Massage Techniques
for Horse and Rider

MASSAGE
TECHNIQUES
for Horse and Rider

Mary W Bromiley

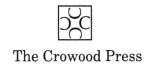

The Crowood Press

First published in 2002 by
The Crowood Press Ltd
Ramsbury, Marlborough
Wiltshire SN8 2HR

www.crowood.com

This impression 2005

British Library Cataloguing-in-Publication Data
A catalogue record for this book is available from the British Library.

ISBN 1 86126 356 2

Photographs and illustrations
Penelope Slattery

Disclaimer
**There are no restrictions for the administration of human therapy, but in the UK
a Parliamentary Act, The Veterinary Act 1996, restricts the treatment of an animal
by any persons other than a qualified veterinary surgeon.**

**Treatment or therapy should only be administered if the veterinary surgeon
normally in charge of the animal has given permission to a therapist who has
been independently contacted by the owner or trainer. To treat or massage without
veterinary permission constitutes a legal offence.**

**It should be clearly understood by anyone practising the techniques described
in this text, that interaction with a body, through the medium of touch, will result
in a series of reactive responses throughout the body's systems, which is why the
treatment is so highly regulated.**

**It is very important to be aware of the risks involved in working with horses and
ponies. Neither the author nor publisher are to be held responsible in any way for
injury sustained by persons who, after reading this book, may practise massage or
any other of the therapies described, neither can they be held responsible for any
adverse effects or injury resulting from the inappropriate use of massage or allied
therapies.**

Typeset by Phoenix Typesetting, Ilkley, West Yorkshire.

Printed and bound in Great Britain by CPI, Bath

Contents

Foreword

My association with Mary Bromiley through her involvement with the New Zealand Three-Day Event Team is without doubt one of the most fortunate encounters of my career.

Learning from Mary and seeing first hand the benefits of massage in maintaining and producing competition horses has enabled me to continue to enjoy success at International level. 'Therapy through touch' has now become an integral part of my daily management routine and I consider that it plays a vital role in the general well-being of my horses, as well as assisting in their preparation, performance and recovery.

Mary is a World leader in equine massage and is also an excellent teacher. We are very lucky that through this book she is prepared to share her considerable knowledge with us in a language that we can all understand.

Blyth Tait MBE

Double World Champion, Olympic Champion, Atlanta, World Ranked No 1 five times, Winner Burghley Horse Trials 2001

Preface

The very word 'massage' requires explanation, as many people only understand it in terms of erotic connotations. Perhaps the most apt and comprehensive definition is 'therapy through touch'.

The object of this text is to enable the reader to identify and understand the reasons and philosophies underlying the various massage techniques currently used as therapy for both horse and rider.

It is hoped that the knowledge gained will enable the aspiring masseur to make an informed choice of the pertinent method for a given situation, rather than relying on random selection.

ACKNOWLEDGEMENTS AND DEDICATION

No book is ever written without some trauma, and this one is no exception. Despite the efforts of 'call Bob', my computer guru, who has tried to make me, a grandmother, understand very simple computer basics, second nature to the five-year-old of today, of my younger daughter Rabbit who has filed, saved and found with unfailing good nature, I managed to have my brief case, containing the first complete text on disc, stolen after the Sydney Olympics. Only the computer knows what I did to lose every thing it had kept safe in its guts till I returned.

So grateful thanks to my family who have put up with my rewriting, especially my eldest daughter Penelope and her camera.

The book must be dedicated to the many horses and riders who have allowed me to work on them, but most especially to the New Zealand Three-Day Event Team, Blyth Tait, Mark Todd, Paul O'Brien, Andrew Nicholson, Vaughan Jefferies, their horses and their grooms, not forgetting Wally Niederer, vet *extraordinaire*.

1999, 2000, 2001, Turks and Caicos Islands, Exmoor.

Introduction

In the Western world the concepts and philosophy fundamental to Oriental medicine are rarely considered by those who aim to adopt the methods and offer therapy based upon the described techniques. There is a common misconception that the methods, centuries old, are easily mastered, and can be practised effectively either by reading a text or attending a weekend seminar.

My own introduction to Oriental medicine occurred in Malaysia and came from a Buddhist monk who was in his tenth year of training; yet he would not be considered safe to practise either massage or acupressure until he had completed a further five years of study. Sent to study the Western medical approach, he was amazed at the inability of the qualified persons he met to 'read' their patients by using hair texture, skin feel, tongue colour or pulse variation, to name but a few of his tools.

He stressed the need, while questioning a patient, for observation, the ability to listen, to smell and to read through touch. These senses, referred to as 'the four methods', are considered as important by those practising Oriental medicine as are the diagnostic tools and machines used by those trained in Western medical schools. A knowledge of *yin* and *yang*, and of the inter-relationship between earth, metal, water, wood and fire, the 'five transformations', must also be considered

before therapy can truly be said to be based on Eastern methods.

Fortunately for those wishing to practise massage, one type of touch technique, and acupressure, another, both have become 'westernized' in concept, but there remains scepticism associated with many of the claims attributed to the methods by those practising Western medicine, this stemming from the fact that only anecdotal suggestion, rather than scientific data, is offered to back the claims of both patients and practitioners.

Regrettably most Western medical teaching has failed, for one reason or another, to accept the interaction between, reliance upon and necessary integration of all the systems comprising the whole. Consideration of the whole is fundamental to Oriental thought in the context of health. The ideas of cause and effect, the fact that all body systems are considered to be inextricably inter-linked and that no individual system can function without the backup of all its fellows, leads to the logical concept that malfunction of any system, or even a part of a system affects the whole; conversely by influencing a system the effects will to a greater or lesser degree affect and benefit the whole.

These fundamental principles and philosophies, upon which Oriental medicine is based, are still largely incomprehensible to the average Western mind, and Western medical science remains for the

8

most part sceptical of the beneficial effects attributed to the use of massage and acu point stimulation. The Western approach has tended to exclude the whole and to focus upon a single effect or reaction without due consideration of the problem in its entirety.

The following example may help to clarify the Western concept. A very charming lady was treated for 'tennis elbow'. Treatment was given and she telephoned a few days later to say all was well. She returned with the same symptoms several weeks later. Treatment was repeated, she reported recovery, only to reappear after several weeks. Shortly after a treatment session, when driving through her village her therapist passed her house and saw her struggling with an 'up and over' garage door. Stopping she enquired if the door was stiff? 'A pig' she was told. The patient complied with the suggestion that the mechanism be oiled. On settling her account she penned 'quite an expensive oil can'! In my view therapy had failed, although the diagnosis was correct and the condition recovered following the appropriate therapy failure occurred due to a confined concept of the problem (Western approach) with no expansion of thought aimed at questioning effectively to establish the cause (Eastern concept). At the first treatment session her lifestyle should have been discussed to identify the cause of her injury.

At least three years of committed study is probably the minimum time required to change a situation of existing pre-indoctrinated Western thought and become able to embrace and identify with the concepts of the wider Oriental approach. Without making this effort to retrain and expand the mind to accept concepts common in Eastern thinking, along with an in-depth appreciation of the complex, intricate inter-linkage of all life systems, it is impossible to choose and execute a responsible therapy plan utilizing Oriental methods.

Massage and all the techniques discussed in the text are associated with touch, a sensation appreciated and recorded via specialist nerve receptors sited within the structural layers of the skin. The 'messages' conceived are immediately, resulting from stimulation of nervous tissue, flashed through out the body.

In 1991 Butler stated, with regard to the nervous system, 'if there is some change in part of the system, then it will have repercussions for the whole'. Returning to the Oriental concept which considers, due to the inter-connection between all parts that together constitute the whole, that by influencing any system or part of a system the whole will be affected, we begin to realize science is beginning to give some credibility and offer proof to enhance the validity of ancient concepts. While many have still to be proven satisfactorily to appease the Western mind the Oriental approach to healing is unlikely to be totally overwhelmed by the chemically reliant systems of today. The growth in popularity and widespread practice of these ancient therapies is not only a reflection of a changing public attitude and general unease regarding the use of man-manufactured chemicals, but is also a testimony to the beneficial effects of these therapies lasting as they have, with little change for over 5,000 years.

This text aims to bridge the gap between East and West by demonstrating the fact that today's diverse 'massage' approaches all have a common origin.

1 Origins of Massage

HISTORICAL BACKGROUND

Massage techniques can, for the purpose of understanding, be divided broadly into two main categories.

In the first category are systems based upon Chinese medical techniques and philosophies. The use of massage was thought to have originated in China, where documentation of the methods date back to around 2,700BC. Chinese medical knowledge was not thought to have spread to the West until considerably later, but there is now evidence to suggest either a much earlier arrival or that the techniques were developed concurrently in countries with similarly advanced civilizations such as Egypt, Persia or Crete. To date, there is no firm evidence to support this other than a possible link through markings on the body of a man found in a glacial melt in 1991.

Carbon dating has determined that the 'Iceman' died in the Neolithic period (c. 3,000BC). The intact body, when revealed by a melting glacier on the Swiss-Italian border in 1991, was found to have marks described and documented at the time as 'tattoos'. These marks have recently been identified as those used in acu treatment for arthritis of the knees and the low back. X-rays and examination of the Iceman's body shortly after discovery, showed him to have suffered, during life, from arthritis of the knees and low back.

This remarkable finding suggests either that knowledge of such techniques had spread from one civilization to another, indicating that people were travelling vast distances far earlier than previously thought, or that these skills were concurrently but independently developed by several civilizations.

In the West, massage is described for the first time around 500BC in the writings of Hippocrates, the Greek physician considered to be the father of Western medicine. In the first century BC, Galen, a Roman physician, wrote at least sixteen books describing the use of massage. One recounts its use for gladiators injured in combat, and is probably the first book relating to, and describing sports massage.

The second category, Western massage, is first described at the beginning of the nineteenth century, when French missionaries carried back to France a Chinese book known as the *Cong Fou*. The medical texts contained in the *Cong Fou*, considered to be the work of Tao-Tse, were translated and adapted to suit French medical practices of that period. Unfortunately, at the time when the French translated the *Cong Fou*, the idea of total body harmony, even the concept of considering the relationship of a diagnosed symptom to the body as a whole, did not fit Western perceptions. Thus the very basis upon which Chinese medicine had been built over centuries was ignored and lost.

It is important to understand that some methods of therapy in the translated texts were devised to suit the conditions prevailing at the time and are not necessarily pertinent today. In some instances even the medical conditions for which treatments were devised either no longer exist, or the methods suggested are no longer, in view of scientific advancement, applicable or useful.

The names used to describe massage techniques may seem confusing – a hotchpotch of languages. This is because the French were the first to translate, record and describe the methods employed by the Chinese. Many of the names adopted by those early translators are still in French, for example *effleurage* and *tapotmente*, although the word massage is derived from the Arabic, meaning 'to press'.

The methods and techniques so described were later to become known as Swedish massage, for it was a Swede, Professor Henrik Ling (1776–1839) who adopted the methods and developed the principles which are still in general use today. The hand techniques he described and taught form the basic methods of delivering all types of massage, whatever the name coined.

Ling also founded an institute in Stockholm, pioneering a system in which massage and movement were combined. This approach was later to become known as medical gymnastics. Whilst the addition of movement steered Ling nearer to the original Chinese concept, the full implications of the approach – a requirement for all the body systems to be in balance – was either not understood by Ling, although he had visited China to study their methods, or was ignored by him, possibly because it proved unacceptable to the contemporary Western thinking.

Although early evidence of the use of massage and acutherapy is to be found in European texts, and the methods were undoubtedly used, over the centuries popularity appears to have declined, other than for the use of Ling's Swedish massage.

The Opium Wars, world wars and internal unrest reduced communication between China and the West, so it was not until the early 1970s, when visitors were allowed into China, that Chinese medicine, and acupuncture in particular, came to the attention of the Western world once again.

CHINESE MEDICINE

Besides being the probable founders of massage, the Chinese were also using local pressure techniques to achieve beneficial body effects. The early medical practitioners were very conscious of the need for balance, not only in living beings, but also between all the natural elements which, together with animals and plants, constitute life in the fullest sense. This requirement for balance is the basis of Chinese philosophy and is also to be found in most other approaches to health documented in ancient Eastern scripts.

Massage was not used solely as a cure, it was also viewed as a means of promoting health – an early form of preventative medicine. The importance attached to the maintenance of good health is demonstrated by the fact that Chinese and other Eastern physicians were only paid if their patients remained healthy!

Before the use of therapy of any sort, the diagnostic procedure would include pulse readings (each individual pulse beat is considered to reveal five different, significant signs) and the balance of the patient's *yin* and *yang*. A full examination was a lengthy process, and even today, if using traditional methods, a consultation takes far longer and is conducted in much greater depth than Western medical examination procedures.

Following diagnosis, by activating energy channels or meridians through massage, it was possible to direct the naturally present body energy of the subject to reinstate balance and so regain health. This energy use was always incorporated within a carefully selected therapy protocol, and utilized in a manner designed to restore harmony within both the mind and body of the subject.

Acupressure, Acupuncture

Moving on in time, stimulation of all systems, comprising the whole body mass, was developed. This was achieved by using selected local 'points', which are still known as acupressure or acupuncture points. Some of today's massage descriptions refer to 'trigger points'. In fact, many are acu points, thus trigger-point massage must be considered as a form of acupressure.

Acupressure preceded acupuncture by at least a thousand years. The eventual supersedence of acupuncture does not appear to have occurred because the results of acupressure were inferior, but because of the class structure prevailing at the time. The respect required to be accorded to those in power, necessitated that the physician touch his patients as little as possible. A method of using acupressure points, without physical contact between patient and physician, had therefore to be devised. Following on, and to avoid the necessity of any 'loss of face' by the patient due to body exposure, 'points' on body extremities such as the ears, fingers, toes, and soles of the feet were developed. Like so many other medical advances, necessity proved to be the mother of invention!

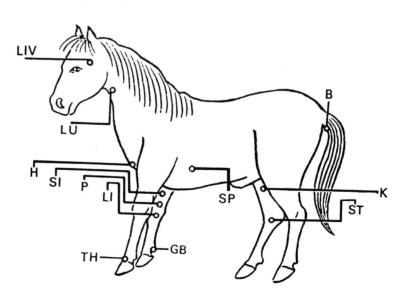

Drawing of a horse showing the location of the 12 meridian points.

LIV–liver, LU–lung, H–heart, P–pericardum, SP–spleen, K–kidney, TH–triple burner, ST–stomach, GB–gall bladder, LI–large intestine, B–bladder, SI–small intestine.

Source: Veterinary Acupuncture. Compiled 100BC

Records of the treatment of animals first appears in a text compiled around 722BC, the *Nei Ching*. While other species such as the camel, the pig and even the chicken are well-endowed with points, early illustrations depicting the horse merely show twelve meridians without specific local points. The main equine illustration used in early texts is said to have been sourced from the *BA Ryo Taizen* text, compiled around 100BC (*see* page 13).

A further complication arose for the early exponents of equine acutherapy: the location of points in man and in other species is very precisely described, all texts identifying point sites by the use of exact measurements. These measurements are taken from clearly identifiable landmarks such as bone prominences, a hairline, skin creases, the eye. Once identified, the distance and direction from the appropriate landmark are described. The distance is measured first in units which correspond to inches, called either *chun*, *tsun*, or *pounce*, dependent upon the text, then in *fen*, these corresponding to 0.1 of an inch.

Nowhere in Chinese texts is there described such a precise measurement protocol for the horse. The only reference states that a *chun*, or *tsun*, is the width of the sixteenth rib at the level of the tuber coxae.

Down the ages and particularly in the twentieth century the horse has been endowed with points, many of which appear to correspond with stress or trigger points described in modern texts.

During the 1970s, there was a growth of interest in the use of acupuncture for pain control in the horse, particularly in the USA. Unfortunately, very little reliable information was available as many of the points pertinent to human and other species, rather than to the horse alone, were included in early equine charts. A further difficulty was presented by the fact that equine skin is very mobile, making exact point location extremely difficult. These factors appear to have caused confusion and dissatisfaction amongst the veterinary profession and their clients, and resulted in a lack of clinical success.

SHIATSU – A JAPANESE CONCEPT

Known originally as *Tao Yinn*, Shiatsu, a name not coined until early in the twentieth century, is compiled from two written characters *shi* (finger) and *atsu* (pressure). The official definition from the Japanese Ministry of Health states that 'Shiatsu is administered by the thumbs, fingers and palms, without the use of any instrument, mechanical or otherwise, to apply pressure to the skin, to correct internal malfunctioning, promote or maintain health and to treat specific diseases'. Western teaching has added the knees, forearms, elbows and feet of the therapist as usable tools.

Shiatsu originated in China and embraces a health approach equivalent to the Chinese concept of the 'whole'. In China, a number of slightly different medical disciplines were developed, each pertinent to the requirements of a particular region – lifestyle, diet, even disease patterns varied widely according to geographical location. Thus it was the traditional methods practised in the regions of China most accessible to Japanese traders that were brought back and adopted in Japan, where we first find them described in Japanese texts around

530BC. As with all Eastern health systems the 'whole' is always considered, and the early *Tao Yinn* features were incorporated within the already present Japanese system, the *Do-In Ankyo.*

Shiatsu is a form of manipulation therapy, the purpose of which is to change, by the use of pressure, the activity not just of the tissues in the area being worked, but also the energy of the body mass and the behaviour of associated organs. The techniques focus on exerting static pressure over described areas of the body activating only the points appropriate both for the problems identified and the body systems involved. Seemingly many of these areas correspond to meridians and acu points.

Rather as Ling later combined movement and massage, Shiatsu also embraced a system of exercises. These exercise routines were combined with personal sensory control through the use of self-massage and self-applied point pressure.

This system was very comprehensive, including and utilizing in its disciplines an extensive range of therapies incorporating not only exercises, but also diet, meditation, manipulation and pressure – this combination was to become collectively known, by the tenth century, as *Anma.* During the *Edo* era, some 300 years ago, aspiring Japanese doctors were made to study *Anma* because of the depth of knowledge of anatomy, structure, energy channels and pressure points the system demanded. *Anma* tuition was not only considered superior to that available in medical schools, but also ensured that an informed choice of appropriate treatment was selected from those available, namely herbs, acupuncture, or medical exercises.

Nowadays, Shiatsu is mainly practised in Western countries, where the methods are seemingly rather more popular than in the country of its origin where the techniques tend to be considered old-fashioned.

15

2 Varied Methodology

Massage was first developed for the human species and, although loosely described by the Greek writer Xenophon in his treatise on horsemanship, until recently there has been little factual information on the transposition of the 'art' (for good massage is an art) from human to horse.

Over recent years massage has become increasingly popular and the benefits are becoming recognized for both horse and rider. The techniques, particularly if the Swedish methods are employed, might be considered by some, as far as the horse is concerned, to be a way of grooming by hand. Watching my own horses and realizing how much they enjoyed the experience, prompted me to explore the various approaches.

SWEDISH MASSAGE

Swedish massage describes and embraces all the classic massage techniques. Every other form of massage utilizes one or more of the Swedish methods of hand or finger application. The strokes are directed, insofar as it is possible, to run in parallel with the flow of two of the body fluids, venous blood and lymph, as they return towards the centre of the body.

Effluerage

The aim of effleurage is to relax the subject and all Swedish massage routines begin and end with this technique. Following effleurage, the choice of massage technique will be determined by the site being worked, tissue depth and mass, and the required end result.

Petrissage

As the underlying tissue relaxes, a variety of methods such as kneading, wringing, picking up, shaking, and deep vibration are employed. All are designed to produce local compression followed by a release, with emphasis directed towards influencing deep tissue.

Tapotment

These techniques comprise light vibration, hacking, clapping, tapping and pounding. They are designed to deliver stimulatory signals to the tissues.

Friction

Friction is a locally applied technique performed by using a single fingertip, or one fingertip reinforced by a second, to irritate underlying tissue by using short, cross-fibre movements.

Sport Massage

The principles of sport massage can be described as the use of classic Swedish massage techniques to prepare the subject for competition, assist during the event, and aid recovery afterwards.

Each equine discipline varies slightly in muscle requirement, both for horse and rider or driver. A masseur should observe and be familiar with the variety of situations encountered by competitors and their mounts. For example, a person driving in a governess cart may be seated in a slightly twisted position, as will a rider on a side-saddle. The muscle usage by the pony pulling the governess cart will vary from that of the horse carrying a side-saddle. The dressage horse and its rider will experience muscle discomfort not apparent in the racehorse. Therefore, the masseur should take careful note of the:

- way each horse moves;
- hazards encountered during competition;
- state of the ground;
- terrain;
- time of day; and
- air temperature.

Such considerations will influence the type and duration of massage, and will also help to select the time when massage will be of most benefit. For instance, in some situations it is sensible to work on the rider first, leaving the horse to relax, cool down, drink and possibly feed.

One thing is certain, no two apparently identical situations will ever be exactly the same. Flexibility of attitude is important as every horse and rider will experience their own individual problems and every subject massaged will react slightly differently. It is therefore essential that those working for clients at competition have massaged the subjects several times previously. Little benefit is gained if a shoulder massage makes the rider feel slightly sick (and this can happen) or a horse becomes so relaxed it fails to give of its best.

CONNECTIVE TISSUE MASSAGE (CTM)

In CTM it is considered possible to influence the autonomic nervous system, in particular the sympathetic division, by working areas overlying certain types of connective tissue described as 'reflex zones'; each is linked to a particular organ or system.

Due to the interaction between organs and superficial reflex zones, stimulation will achieve a widespread effect. This interaction has been described in many scholarly papers, all of which support the concept that the body functions as a whole, whilst acknowledging that there is still a lack of understanding regarding the complexity of the reflex interactions present throughout a body. Interaction was considered to be neural but specialist cell messengers and chemical signals have recently been identified and recognized as transmitting media, thus providing a scientific reason for the success attributed to an age-old method.

17

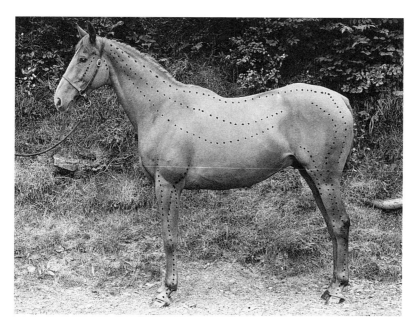

*Zone lines.
It is interesting to observe the zones mirror the position of some meridians and anatomically described lymphatic drainage channels.*

Many hypotheses have been made as to the reasons for the benefits reported following stimulation of the connective tissue matrix. Rolf (1997) suggested that changes in the ground substance of the connective tissue matrix occur following pressure. First there is a change in the viscosity of the natural gel, resulting in a piezoelectric effect; then, as the pressure is removed, the tissues return to their previous neutral state. Changes in tissue state, wherever they occur, are known to be multi-layered: any gross reconstruction or change will produce subcellular, molecular, regenerative responses.

While links between superficial points and organs are believed to exist, and the evidence would indicate that this is the case, lack of scientific investigation makes it impossible to verify. In a paper published in 1996, Giniaux produced a series of possible links between superficial points and organs in the horse (*see* Appendix I). It should, however, be emphasized that

these are no more than suggestions.

There are questions to be asked and issues to address before embarking on CTM. It should be remembered that those practising any form of therapy in China and Japan have been trained to examine their subjects in a medical context, thus making an informed diagnosis.

The masseur must ask himself:

- which zone influences which system or organ?
- does that organ or system require stimulation?
- will massage do more harm than good? (In man, recorded adverse reactions include palpitations, fainting, vomiting and emotional release.)

While the technique is described in many texts and is offered for the horse, the author suggests that it is not safe or suitable for general use, unless sanctioned by a doctor or veterinarian following a diagnostic procedure.

LYMPHATIC DRAINAGE

The body's lymphatic system is concerned with defence. The system manufactures lymphocytes, specialist cells designed to combat invasion of the body by organisms and to remove toxic material or waste.

Under normal conditions, lymphatic fluid is contained within the lymphatic vessels – a comprehensive network of small tubes and tubules resembling and running in parallel with those of the venous system. These vessels have special valves that ensure unidirectional fluid flow. All the vessel complexes interconnect to areas of specialist tissue known as glands or lymph nodes.

As a result of certain specific conditions, the lymphatic system may cease to maintain its normal fluid flow, causing massive swelling (oedema) in the affected region. This condition usually affects a single limb. Those who have viewed the condition in a horse will remember the vast distension created in the affected limb with the skin stretched to its limit, often oozing fluid. In man, the affected area should be positioned to allow gravitational drainage, which, coupled with specialist massage, can be very effective.

Unlike most massage routines, which are commonly performed by starting in those areas furthest from the central body mass and working inward, lymphatic massage starts centrally. This is necessary to ensure that the vessels at the core of the system are cleared before even more fluid is forced centrally towards an already overloaded area. Massage is then performed over the adjoining distal segment and continued by working each distal segment in a manner that ensures fluid is encouraged to migrate into a 'cleared' segment.

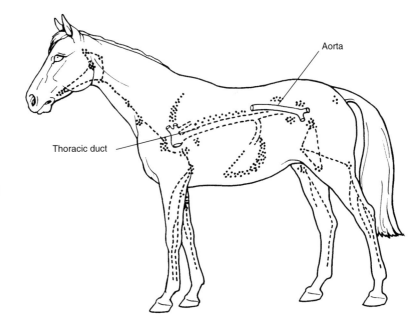

Main lymphatic channels and gland masses. All lie deep within the body mass.
•*• = lymph nodes*
--- *= main lymphatic channels*

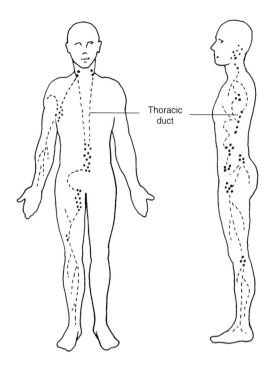

Main lymphatic channels and gland masses. All lie deep within the body mass but those sited in the neck, armpit and groin are palpable when swollen.
••• = *lymph nodes*
--- = *main lymphatic channels*

Thoracic duct

It is important to note the following when performing lymphatic drainage:

- The areas worked should conform to the described anatomical course of the lymph channels.
- Due to the skin tension, all techniques used for manual lymphatic drainage should be performed in a stationary manner.
- Skin slide must be avoided, thus the technique is one of light pressure with the hands exerting an inward compression, being lifted and re-applied.

The lymphatic system of the horse is very poorly described in anatomy texts – the location and extent of vessels in the limbs are rarely documented. The clusters of lymph nodes appear to be sited deep within the tissues. Postural drainage is impossible – however, in cases of massive oedema, massage does sometimes appear to be of benefit but only if there is no infection present as lymph can spread infection to other areas remote from the primary site.

Sport Lymphatic Drainage

There are exponents of sport lymphatic drainage for the horse. In natural situations, the mild tension forces engendered by minor muscle contractions, created as the animal moves while grazing or wandering from one area to another, influence the lymphatic and venous vessels, aiding fluid flow within by the creation of a compression and release phenomenon. This compression followed by release is transmitted to the vessels, acting in a manner comparable to a soft-walled tube being mechanically squeezed and freed in order to force fluid through its length.

Due to the confines imposed by stabling, the horse is unable to cleanse its systems as it would under natural conditions. Lymphatic drainage assists the removal of waste toxins as both lymph and venous blood flow act as transporters.

CRYOTHERAPY

The use of cryotherapy is confined to recent soft tissue injury. The application of ice, iced or cold towels will help to prevent excessive swelling in an area damaged by collision with an obstacle, a kick or a fall. Ice massage is therefore a useful procedure at competition.

The massage technique should consist of circular movements – the ice or iced towel moved slowly with minimal pressure over the area of damage. The physiological effects will be apparent after approximately 15–20 minutes. Massage should then stop for 20–30 minutes before another 15–20 minute session is given.

Do not overdo ice – too much can be as unproductive as too little.

UNDERWATER MASSAGE

Underwater massage, using purpose-created water 'wellie' boots filled with iced water, is the most effective method of treating soft tissue injuries of the limbs, both equine and human.

Masseurs should note that damaged bone, such as a stress or complete fracture, reacts unfavourably to excessive cold. The pain experienced by the subject often apparently increasing to intolerable levels as the effects of the cold diminish.

ACUPRESSURE AND ACUPUNCTURE

The manipulation of energy in order to achieve body harmony and balance within all systems, is the governing principle behind the theories associated with acupressure and acupuncture. For years the existence of acu points has been discussed: reviled as total nonsense by some, accepted by others. Recent electro-physiological studies of the skin have demonstrated areas of decreased electrical resistance at traditional point sites.

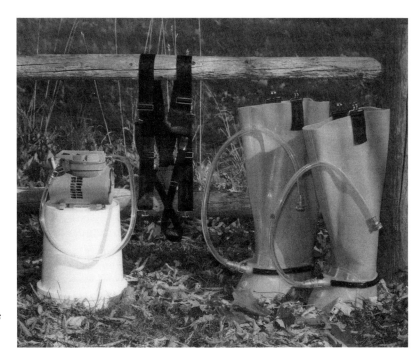

Specially made 'wellie' boots are very effective for helping soft-tissue damage to the limbs of both horse and rider.

21

In addition, very recent histologic research has demonstrated small micro-tubules penetrating fascia at sites where acu points are said to be located. These tubules, besides possessing a prolific micro-circulation, appear also to be richly endowed with free nerve endings.

For many reasons, not least that of possible infection which is always a hazard in non-sterile conditions, acupressure is the natural method of choice when considering the horse. It is also a preferable approach for the human in non-sterile situations.

Traditional Chinese medicine describes twelve meridians in both man and horse, each relating to a specific organ or system. Both species are also endowed with other named points, each with a specific functional importance. By stimulation of appropriate points it is considered possible to influence the natural flow of energy along the line or path of each meridian. This theory corresponds neatly with the beneficial effects described and associated with the 'reflex zone' stimulation of CTM.

At acu points, the energy force is located close to the body surface, allowing externally applied pressure stimuli to be effective.

Four types of neural structures are considered to be influential and for the sake of clarity are described as follows:

Type 1　Considered to be sited at motor points. Anatomically, a motor point describes the area within a muscle housing the motor nerve ending or command cell. Motor points correspond to trigger points.

Type 2　Considered to be sited in the superficial nerve complexes found in the sagital plane along the upper (dorsal) and ventral mid-lines.

Type 3　Correspond to superficial, previously identified sites, recognized as housing high-density nerve plexi.

Type 4　Found at musculo-tendinous junctions where the golgi sensor is present.

Note: The UK Veterinary Act does not allow any person to use needles on any form of livestock, unless permission has been obtained from a qualified veterinary surgeon.

STRESS AND TRIGGER POINT MASSAGE

Stress point massage may be used as a method of relieving muscle fatigue but is of greater use if localized areas of tension have been identified, these probably secondary to actual tissue damage rather than plain fatigue.

Anatomically, stress or *ashi* points tend to be located approximately two-thirds of the way along a muscle. Muscles change their tissue architecture as they near the area where they insert. The segment of change, described as the musculo-tendinous junction is richly supplied with neural sensors. Thus stimulation of stress or *ashi* points will engender a greater generalized effect than that achieved or even required by the use of conventional massage.

The experienced masseur will usually give a general body massage, or massage the fatigue areas pertinent to the discipline, reassessing the tension area after massage. If local tension is still present, it may be appropriate to work the stress or *ashi* points of the area. In the case of horses, the agreement of a veterinary surgeon must first be secured.

THE BOWEN TECHNIQUE

A comparative newcomer to the range of techniques on offer is that developed in Australia by Tom Bowen (1902–1982) and appropriately named the Bowen Technique. The method was documented in the 1970s by Oswald Rentch, an osteopath who worked with Bowen towards the end of his life.

No scientific research or explanation for the undoubted success of Bowen's methods is currently available. Bowen claimed that the touch methods he advocated rebalanced and released already present energy, allowing the body to utilize its own repair mechanisms.

The Bowen method is one of light touch. The thumb pads or fingertips are applied over the body surface in a manner that moves or rolls slack skin overlying areas of tissue tension in a predetermined pattern. The pressure applied needs to ensure enough contact with the skin to avoid slipping or sliding but to be sufficient to achieve the 'roll'. This movement creates secondary stimulation to the complex of nerve endings (neural receptors) in the underlying fascia.

The results claimed and methods of applying the Bowen Technique mirror, to a degree, those described for CTM and meridian stimulation, although the purists of each might well disagree.

AROMATHERAPY

In a natural environment animals depend upon a highly developed sense of smell both for recognition and survival. In domesticated species, these have often been exploited by man – the truffle-hunting pig and the tracker dog are just a couple of examples.

Modern man no longer needs to rely on his olfactory sense for survival, and the sense of smell among the general population is probably less well developed than in the past. However, with some natural sensitivity and practice, the sense can be heightened and developed to detect very subtle variations in smell – perfumery experts, for example.

The olfactory organ, which receives and analyzes smells, is sited in the nose, housed within the nasal mucosa on the roof of the upper area of the nasal cavity.

It is probable that one of the earliest methods of using fragrances was through the burning of incense. The Egyptians appear to have been amongst the first to use this method – a symbol, frequently depicted on the walls of ancient temples and tombs, shows smoke lines rising from a semicircular, handled object. Frankincense, myrrh, cinnamon and sandalwood were prized commodities. All true perfumes today are made by distillation, an art unknown to the Egyptians who soaked plant material in a prepared oil, often olive oil, to create their fragrances. The usage of fragrance is described in many cultures for a wide range of applications including medicine, exorcism, religion and divination.

In early writings, aromatherapy is frequently described as 'therapy using scents or odours', which suggests that aromatherapy does not necessarily utilize massage as the primary source of delivery. Today, however, aromatherapy is understood to be the use of massage with essential oils. The skin is a porous membrane and suitably prepared, fragrant and non-fragrant preparations are able to filtrate through the skin, be absorbed into the underlying capillary network and achieve the desired effect.

It is worth noting that natural chemicals in some plant distillations contain substances which, when absorbed by the body, have effects similar to substances prohibited at competition. Some are stimulatory, others have a sedative effect.

TELLINGTON TOUCH EQUINE AWARENESS METHOD (TTEAM)

When compared with the antiquity of the Oriental approach to health maintenance, TTEAM is a very recent technique. The methods used and activities incorporated are the result of years of study by Linda Tellington Jones.

In the 1960s she became interested in equine massage, then moved on to study the Feldenkrais method of human body work. This is an approach based on the concept that pain can create secondary problems, both physical and mental. However, this can be avoided and health restored by achieving balance of the body systems through selectively applied touch techniques combined with exercises.

Once again we are returning to ideas similar to those of Ling with his development of medical gymnastics, and to the age-old concept of creating a method to address the whole rather than the particular.

Linda Tellington Jones has shown that the interaction between exercises and her method of Ttouch (or specialist massage techniques), achieves expansion of a horse's general awareness – a sense that has been restricted by domestication. The technique also improves balance, coordination, and trust.

The lines described by Ttouch practitioners as areas for stimulation in the horse are comparable to the reflex zones described by the advocates of CTM in the human as are the methods of finger/hand application (*see* page 18).

3 The Aspiring Masseur

HAND EDUCATION

For those who intend to use massage regularly or train for a career in massage, it is essential to make time for hand education. It is sensible to try to incorporate hand education into day-to-day activities, as few people, however good their original intention, will find the time to practise daily. It must be continued until interactions, sensory input, and communication between the hands and the body surface begin to automatically impart information. After all, the hands are the 'tools of the trade'.

The techniques described in the text can be easily learnt, given time and practice. A sensible approach is to learn to use your hands by working on a friend rather than trying to start to learn on a horse. The reason for this is that the friend can describe the sensations your hands are delivering which will enable you to identify, by incorporating tactile recognition with voice information, the feelings he or she receives from your hands, and those you record through your hands as they perform the delicate operation of tissue moulding. Having someone to talk to is also useful because it forces you to breathe. Beginners tend to hold their breath as they strain to 'get it right'. This leads to shoulder tension, which causes rapid fatigue in the hands and arms. While working, try to get some feedback on the following points:

- Are both hands moulding and conforming evenly to the contours of the body?
- Is the contact through palms only, or are the fingers also achieving full contact?
- How much pressure is he or she experiencing through the hands?
- Is the pressure felt equally from both right and left hands?
- Do both hands impart similar sensations?
- Is there a sensation of rhythm or do the techniques feel jerky?

The horse cannot communicate thus and mistakes with a horse often lead to loss of confidence and irritation on both sides.

Another requirement is to learn to appreciate or 'read' the condition of the body upon which you are working. Through practice, you will learn to interpret the sensations received through your hands as they connect with the outer surface of the body. The depth and content of this information will increase with time as sensitivity improves.

As a masseur you must learn to sense not only the state of the tissues lying beneath the skin (do they feel tense, relaxed, warm, cold?), but also indications of general health through the feel of the skin or, in the horse, the coat texture. In former times, doctors felt the hair of their patients – a silky feel indicated the person was in better health than if their hair felt dry. Learn to ask yourself, as you massage:

- How would I be feeling if I had been in a similar situation to this rider and horse?
- Where might I feel stiff?
- Which joints were over-stretched?
- Which muscles might be painful?
- Where and which are the structures involved, relevant to the body surface?

It is not until you are able to make a mental pictorial map of the body, linked to both body movement and its anatomy, along with a well-developed technique of tactile discrimination, that you will become fully effective as a masseur (*see* Chapter 5 Comparative and Surface Anatomy).

Tactile Recognition

Before attempting to massage, it is well worth testing your powers of tactile recognition. If these are poor, they will need to be developed as a masseur requires 'eyes' in the tips of the fingers.

Lesson 1
Collect a series of identical paired objects, each pair should be of a different shape and texture and offer a different resistance when compressed or squeezed. The reason for paired objects is because both hands require equal education, and must interlink so that right follows left in an identical manner in all double-handed techniques.

With eyes closed, feel and identify the individual paired objects. Mentally record shape, texture and resistance to compression, comparing these with a familiar tactile sensation. For example, for those regularly involved with horses: do the objects feel firm like a leather saddle flap or the trace of a driving harness (muscle in spasm); soft like a wool or gel numnah (a relaxed muscle); or hard like an iron or bit (underlying bone)? The mind becomes considerably more focused if the eyes are closed, and tactile recognition will be learnt rapidly.

Lesson 2
Once you have practised general identification, take a pair of objects, perhaps two oranges, and squeeze alternately – first with one hand, then the other. Finally, work both hands simultaneously. Next, try to achieve a state of controlled alternation – as one hand increases contact pressure, the other releases.

Learn to achieve a rhythm between the hands, remembering that massage can be sedative or relaxing, when slow monotonous rhythms are used, or stimulatory by the employment of rapid hand motions.

Lesson 3
After several sessions handling the differing objects, by which time both hands should have imprinted for immediate awareness, try to establish recall so that when massaging the sensation from your hands tells you where you are on the body surface, and what structure lies below. While learning the sensation from an orange suggests a relaxed muscle, a Granny Smith apple, muscle tension. The

edge of a cup imparts a feel similar to that experienced as hands encounter super-ficial bone ridge – a subtly different sensation from that experienced when feeling an apple. Differences between rough and smooth, rounded, curved, and flat also need to be appreciated.

Variations in temperature are import-ant – in the horse, such differences are often both very local and very subtle. The temperature of a horse's lower leg should be similar to the feel of a mug that has been in a refrigerator. Feeling the outer surface of a mug filled with water of various temperatures is a good way of developing heat discrimination.

Muscle Control

It is essential to achieve independent control of the fingers, thumbs and palms during activity and relaxation. Dexterity is also required. Whilst gripping is not a feature of massage, strength in all parts of the hand is necessary.

When first learning to massage, few people will have developed the correct hand musculature to enable them to be really effective. The thumb and little finger each possess their own specialist muscles, which can be identified by turning the hands palms upward. Those of the thumb form a mass, easily recogniz-able if the thumb is moved across the hand towards the little finger. The muscles in the little finger are visible if the finger, working alone, is moved upward away from the palm. The activated muscles create a ridge running from the base of the little finger to the junction of hand to wrist (*see* the illustrations on page 28). Some massage techniques require the tissue mass being worked to be lifted while held

between these two muscle groups, rather than squeezed by the whole hand.

The muscle groups controlling the fingers are sited in the forearm, lying between the wrist and elbow. By the time the muscles have reached the wrist there has been a change in tissue construction, the fibre pattern alignment changing from muscle to tendon.

The muscle groups, acting through their tendons, bend the fingers to the palm of the hand (flexion) and straighten the fingers (extension). Two sets of muscles are responsible for flexion, one set for exten-sion. The ability of these muscles to work the fingers is enhanced by the presence of the interosseous muscles, little feather-like muscles sited between the individual bones forming the basic architecture of the palms of the hands. These small muscles can also spread and close the fingers.

Muscle Strengthening

It is important to emphasize that increased work ability, following on from strengthening exercises, is not instanta-neous. It will take at least six months for untutored hands to strengthen, mould effectively and develop sufficient tactile ability to impart constant, useful messages and information.

Grip and general hand strength can be improved either by squeezing a tennis ball or using a proprietary hand exerciser, available from most sports shops. A strong rubber band or bands, placed around the fingers so that resistance is encountered as they spread, will load and strengthen the interossei. Greatest resistance will be achieved if the rubber bands are sited at the tips of the fingers.

Suppleness within muscle groups is

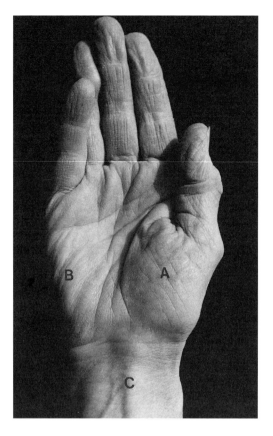

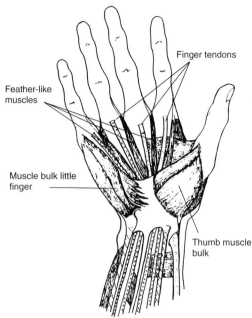

Left and above: *The palmar surface of the hand.*

A   *muscles of the thumb*
B   *muscles of the little finger*
C   *tendon involved in flexing the fingers*

as essential as strength, so stretching and relaxation must be incorporated within any hand education programme. It is possible to create tension in the hands by simulating a hard grip, which should then be followed by a release of tension until the hands feel soft and, if waved gently, flop like a rag doll.

There are a significant number of people who possess hyper-mobile joints. All the joints in the body are capable of an extended range of movement due to ligament laxity. As muscles work in partnership with ligaments to achieve joint stability, it is essential for anyone with the condition to pay particular attention to strengthening the musculature of

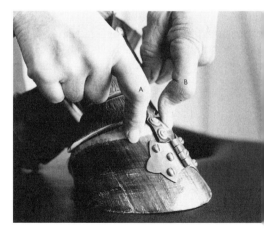

A *Finger is in a neutral position and cannot be damaged.*
B *Finger is hyperextended at the last joint.*

their fingers, hands and arms before attempting to massage, as this condition can lead to injury when massaging, particularly for local techniques using a fingertip.

BODY AWARENESS

Massage becomes exhausting if the masseur is tense. In the beginner, this may be caused by either mental or physical tension – or a combination of the two. Even the experienced masseur may, on occasion, experience tension. If this is the case then no attempt should be made to massage.

When working, the masseur is required to stand, arms held forward of the body. For the inexperienced, this arm position tends to fix the shoulders, creating tension that is relayed down the arms to the hands, achieving rigidity rather than softness. As previously mentioned, shoulder tension has a secondary, respiratory effect – a fixed upper chest (thorax) reduces the ability to breathe efficiently. Reduced oxygen uptake leads to rapid muscle fatigue.

Shoulders and arms should be kept 'soft'. If increased pressure is required to influence deep-sited tissue, this should be generated by the subtle use of body weight rather than energy-consuming dynamic thrusts.

The body weight of the masseur should be balanced over the feet, which should be spread comfortably to achieve easy weight transference between them. The feet may be placed either parallel, or one slightly in advance of the other to allow the upper body to assume a position which achieves:

- economy of balance (reduction of masseur fatigue);
- visualization of the subject (essential to read body language); and
- body weight advantage (reduction of shoulder tension).

PROFESSIONALISM

Despite the fact that in contemporary society, professionalism tends to be the exception rather than the rule, a responsible and meticulous approach to massage is essential for many reasons, not least of which is the threat of malpractice. To avoid any risk of litigation, all masseurs must ensure that:

- When working with a horse, the client's veterinarian has been informed. If any form of treatment by massage is proposed, permission from the client's veterinarian is legally required in the UK.
- When working on a person, a letter should be written or some form of communication made with the client's doctor. This is not a legal requirement, rather a matter of good sense and courtesy.
- Protection is provided by adequate liability insurance.
- Comprehensive, in-depth notes should always be kept (*see* page 153–4).

A liability form to safeguard the masseur, preferably drawn up by a lawyer specializing in equine affairs (*see* Association of Equine Legal Practitioners, Useful Addresses), should be signed by the client before any type of massage is given. The form should be in duplicate, the client holding one copy, the masseur the other. The masseur's copy should be kept with the horse's notes lest, at some future date, there should be some dispute regarding the therapy given.

APPROPRIATE DRESS AND HYGIENE

- Wear a kennel coat, boots or shoes with non-slip soles (not trainers) when working with a horse.
- Nails should be short and clean.
- It is inadvisable to wear jewellery or protruding rings.
- Hair, if long, should be tied back. A cap is useful in a stable or when working outside in the wind.
- When working on a human subject it is particularly important that high standards of personal hygiene are maintained as most massage techniques involve working at close quarters to the client.

It must be remembered that animals have a very acute sense of smell. Colts, even some geldings, particularly those with 'rig' tendencies, can become very unsettled if the masseur has just worked on a filly who was in season; is wearing a provocative deodorant or scent; or if female is herself menstruating. In a situation when, whatever the reason, the horse will neither relax nor remain sufficiently calm for massage to be safe or effective, it is far more responsible not to massage, but to try again another time. Similarly, massage should be abandoned if the masseur is unable to relax.

VISITING YARDS

Most big yards work to routine – mucking out, feeding, exercising and allowing the horses to relax after exercise at more or less the same time each day. Horses appreciate routine, and trying to give a massage if the horse knows it is nearly feed time or the yard is busy, is impossible. If working in a new yard, the masseur should become familiar with and try to fit into the routine, so that massage sessions can take place when the yard is not full of bustle and noise.

In a racing yard the head lad is even more important than the trainer – liaise with him. In an event or livery yard there is usually a senior groom who can be consulted. With the single horse client, arrange a time, be punctual, advise the amount of time required for the massage and respectfully request that they leave you in peace – nothing is more frustrating than the client coming in to see how you are 'getting on' when you have just got a horse to relax. The horse will immediately lose concentration, tense up and swing around towards the familiar voice. It is impossible to give a good massage under such circumstances.

Most clients prefer their horse to be massaged in its own box. However, a wash box, particularly if the weather is cold, and the box equipped with sun and heat lights makes a good alternative.

If this is the first time you have massaged the horse, as much information as possible should be obtained. Details of name, age, colour, sex, discipline etc. should be noted down on the record sheet (*see* Appendix II). Ask questions if insufficient information has been provided, particularly regarding the horse's way of going as this may help to identify areas that require attention. Enquire whether the animal is:

- cold backed;
- stiff when first walked out, relaxing after a period of time;
- stiff on one rein;
- going disunited;
- leaning;

- lacking engagement;
- unable to counter canter;
- crossing its jaw; or
- running down its fences.

If making a return visit to a large yard, make certain the horse in question has not changed boxes – one dark bay TB or grey Welsh pony looks very like another! Check your notes with the appropriate person, there may be some useful information that you may not have been given when the appointment was made, or things may have changed since a previous visit. The date of a race or competition may have altered which will result in a change to the preparation routine. Perhaps, with luck, the horse has improved since its last massage!

Box Preparation

As personal safety is a number one priority, double-check that everything is in order before starting to massage, and never rush. For safety, a horse should always be restrained while being worked upon. This is now law for employees under EU safety rules. Before commencing the massage ensure that you:

- Catch and halter the horse.
- Tie up with a lead rope or shank, making certain there is a breakable loop of twine either between the rope and the D ring, or between the tie ring in the wall and the rope.
- Remove any floor hazards over which you or the horse might fall, for example a feed bowl, salt lick or toy. Remember that horses are easily alarmed if something unusual or frightening occurs, such as the

masseur falling or tripping. Their fright, fight, flight reflex kicks in automatically. There are a number of recorded cases of human death following stable accidents caused by unrestrained animals panicking.

- Skip out the box, removing droppings. Leave the banks but make certain the areas on which the horse will stand are as level as is possible. Unlike massaging a person, who can fully relax their muscles by lying down or partially relax by sitting, the horse has to remain in the standing position and resist gravity, whilst maintaining its balance and trying to relax the area being massaged in response to the neural signals delivered by the hands of the masseur. Some horses turn their heads, either to rest on the masseur's shoulder while their neck is being worked or to try to nibble, as in self-grooming, or when standing head to tail with a companion for mutual grooming. They may automatically rest a hind leg for hind quarter massage, or can be taught to do so.
- Put tools used to 'make good' either outside the box making certain they are not in the way of others, or put them away.
- If the animal is rugged, take them off if it is warm. Quarter the horse if it is cold.
- Make certain the belly straps are either tied or folded over, so they cannot trail or flap against a leg.

After completing the massage, replace the rug and let the horse down, leaving everything exactly as you found it including returning the halter used to its rightful hook or peg. Bring your notes up to date before starting the next case.

Body Language

Never forget to 'read' the horse from the moment you walk into its box until the moment you leave. Apprehension causes the horse to:

- tense up;
- try to move away;
- pull back;
- lay back its ears;
- tuck the tail tight;
- kick; and
- bite angrily rather than giving a 'thank you' lipping or a nibble.

The following features will be observed in a relaxed animal:

- head and neck dropping down;
- ears relaxed;
- the upper eyelid drooping;
- lower lip drooping;
- resting one or other hind leg (with luck the one being worked);
- slow respiration; and
- in the male, dropping the penis.

Position yourself when working on the horse so that you can always watch, or are able to glance easily at, the head. It is from a change of expression that you will get your warning signs. To keep looking at the horse's head is as important as continually checking your rear mirror when driving a car.

RIDER MASSAGE

In an ideal world, the masseur should carry a portable couch, clean towels, a light blanket and at least one pillow. These can either be kept in the centre of the couch when it is folded for easy transportation, or carried in a squashy bag (see the accompanying photo). Trying to make a couch from straw or shaving bales covered with a rug is far from satisfactory for while it is possible to get the client reasonably comfortable, there is almost no way to achieve a working height which will not stress the back of the masseur. The couch can, if there is not a room available, be put up in the tack room, a spare box, or solarium if the yard is so equipped. The Jockey Club's 'Flying Physios', when working at racecourses with jockeys, are usually to be found in the weighing room laundry!

As everyone should know, an effective massage is only possible if the client is comfortable and relaxed. The shoulders and neck can be massaged with the client sitting, but there is still some postural tone present so full relaxation is not possible.

It is difficult to work effectively through clothes but, due to lack of privacy and cold temperatures in winter, minimal clothing-removal must sometimes suffice.

As with horses, it is essential that comprehensive, in-depth notes are taken and maintained (see Appendix II). Time can be saved by making new notes,

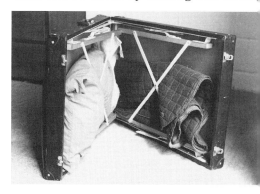

The masseur should carry a portable couch. A towel, blanket and pillow can be kept in the centre when it is folded.

or updating old ones, while the client is getting ready for their massage.

Competition

At a competition, the table in the living quarters of a lorry, provided it is a strong one, converts to a couch of reason-able height. A copy of the competition timetable is a must for the masseur, for it is only when the timetable has been studied that suitable times can be selected to work on riders and their horses. It is important to note the time at which the rider has to be ready and mounted. Remember it takes longer to get ready for dressage than the cross-country phase.

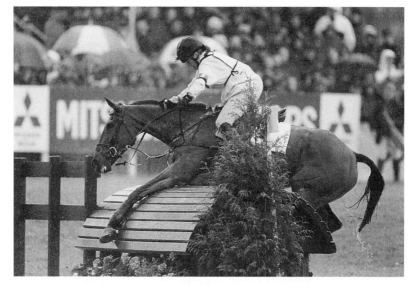

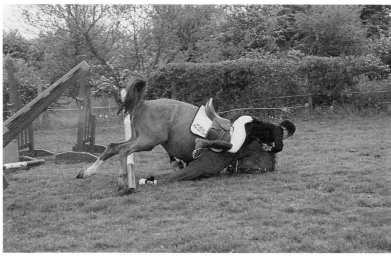

Watch the monitor – the task of identi-fying trauma is much easier if you have seen the fall.

Watch the monitor if possible – should a team member or individual for whom you are working have a fall or refusal, the task of targeting the traumatized areas is far easier when horse and rider return to the stables if the incident has been viewed (*see* the photos on page 33).

Working for a team does not end with riders and horses – the grooms, often exhausted and tense, may need help. Vets, owners, trainers, even *Chefs d'Equippe* have been known to seek help from a team masseur.

Due to endless rule changes and local regulations the masseur should, when working at competition, always check with the official vet to ensure they are allowed to massage. At Badminton Horse Trials, for example, masseurs can only work if they have been signed in by the senior veterinary surgeon.

4 Understanding Anatomy

Anatomy is the term used to describe the architecture of any living thing, be it plant or animal. Conceptual understanding is of mass, experience/education allowing recognition and identification of the exterior of the mass by vision or, in the case of the blind, through touch. Smell or scent are included in the recognition process. The masseur must develop three-dimensional thought, realizing that the mass upon which they work consists of systems, each system built by the clumping of myriad specialist individual cells. The masseur must also comprehend that each cell possesses not only a predestined programme for living and dying, but also the ability to communicate with every other cell in the entire mass. Thus stimulation of one group of cells achieves a wide-ranging effect.

To illustrate this and make it easier to understand, consider an individual with an allergy to bees. The effects following a bee sting in a susceptible person are not, unless an antidote is available, confined to one locality within the body – a general reaction occurs.

Therefore, a basic understanding of the gross composition of and interaction within the structures of the bodies of both man and the horse is necessary for the practice of successful massage and allied techniques.

Simplistically, just like a building, the body is built around a frame. The skeleton, composed of individual bones, forms this frame. All the other components, described as systems, are arranged around, upon, and within the frame. Each and every one of the systems interrelate and interlink. In man and the horse all the body systems are contained within the outermost system, the skin. Just like a building, the body requires efficient fuel, electrical and communication systems, waste disposal facilities, an efficient method of temperature control, a water supply, and constant maintenance and repair.

For the masseur, the following systems are important in both man and horse, and must be appreciated and understood.

SKIN

The skin is the largest body system and covers the entire outer surface of all living beings. It has a very complex structure and is in constant communication with all other body systems. The surface of both the human and equine body have been neurologically mapped to identify areas of sensory perception. These areas of cutaneous enervation, known as dermatomes, are serviced by individual nerve roots.

In man, pain from deep structures is often segmentally referred, that is, pain

35

Right: *Cellular arrangement in the skin to achieve tension bands for added support.*

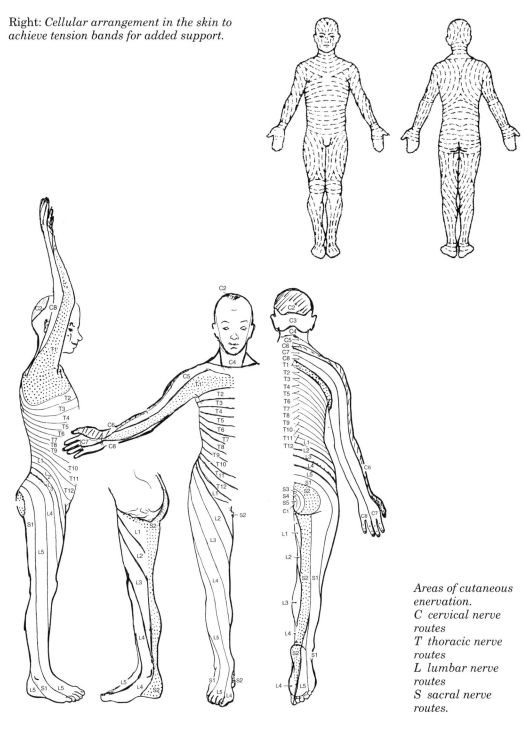

Areas of cutaneous enervation.
C cervical nerve routes
T thoracic nerve routes
L lumbar nerve routes
S sacral nerve routes.

The dermatomes of the horse are not described as being attributed to a single nerve root.

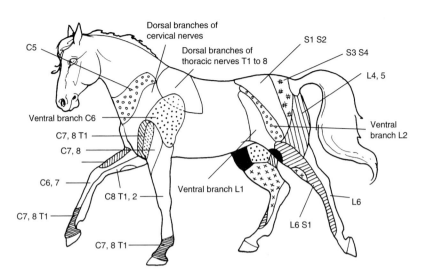

perception is experienced, on the body surface, in the dermatome serviced by the nerve recording from the pain source. A typical example is pain felt in the leg of man when there is a disc pressing on a nerve root in the back. (*See* the picture on page 36.) Man can inform the masseur, the horse cannot; but in the horse the tactile reaction of the skin (cutaneous reflex) is disturbed, often absent if a nerve root is compromized. (*See* the diagram above.) With reference to a neuro anatomy book it is possible to identify structures, particularly muscles, supplied by the nerve supplying the affected dermatome.

The cells of the skin are laid down in a manner that produces tension lines, and so improves support function. In man, skin thickness varies between 0.5 and 3mm, the thickest areas being found on the soles of the feet, the thinnest at the upper eyelids. In the horse, skin thickness varies between 1 and 5mm, being thickest on the upper (dorsal) area of the tail and at the area of mane attachment. As in man, the skin is arranged in a manner that improves support function, these lines are demonstrated by the angles of the hair lie and hair vortices or whorls. The term 'thin-skinned' horse is misleading as the actual skin is not thinner, rather the animal has a heightened sensitivity to external stimuli. The hair on such animals is usually very fine. A horse's skin is sometimes incorrectly described as a 'coat'. In fact the hairs of the human skin and those of the equine coat arise within the architecture of, and are considered to be, an integral part of the skin.

Three-dimensional visualization of the skin is descriptively impossible, even pictorial representation does not mirror the real thing. A visit to a local abattoir to look at the skin on a dead horse is the only way to appreciate fully the minute thickness of the skin, despite its complexity, and to actually visualize the manner in which it attaches to the underlying tissues.

Functions of the Skin

- Communicates with both the external environment and the internal

37

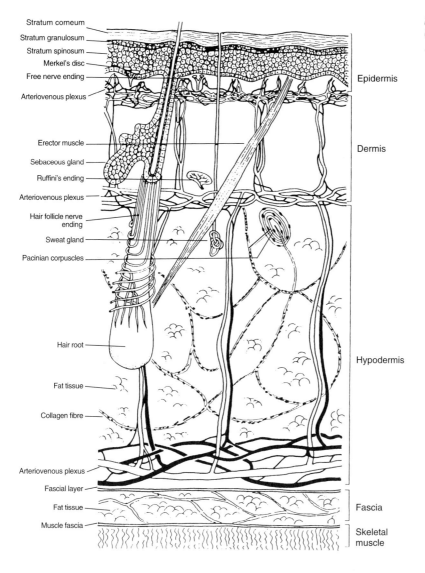

Stratum corneum
Stratum granulosum
Stratum spinosum
Merkel's disc
Free nerve ending
Arteriovenous plexus

Epidermis

Erector muscle
Sebaceous gland
Ruffini's ending
Arteriovenous plexus
Hair follicle nerve ending
Sweat gland
Pacinian corpuscles

Dermis

Hair root

Fat tissue

Collagen fibre

Hypodermis

Arteriovenous plexus
Fascial layer
Fat tissue
Muscle fascia

Fascia

Skeletal muscle

Skin thickness:
0.5–3mm in man,
1–5mm in the horse.

body systems via specialist nerve endings. There is particular involvement in the sensation of touch.

- Acts, particularly in the horse, as a temperature regulator through the raising and lowering of the hairs.
- Sweating and vasodilation.
- Interacts in response to external pain stimulation.

- Acts to prevent dehydration by controlling body fluid loss.
- Uses glands associated with hair follicles to excrete waste products.
- Produces, in association with sunlight, vitamin D.
- Provides a source of antigen presentation to T-lymphocytes.
- Acts as a protective barrier against

38

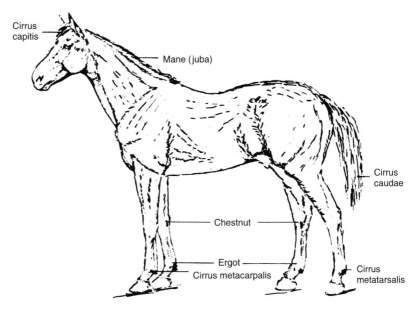

Diagramatic lateral view of a horse showing hair streams representing underlying tension lines of the skin.

Cirrus capitis

Mane (juba)

Cirrus caudae

Chestnut

Ergot

Cirrus metacarpalis

Cirrus metatarsalis

physical injury, poisonous substances and harmful micro-organisms.

Anatomy of the Skin

The skin consists of two distinct layers – the epidermis and the dermis.

The epidermis is the outermost layer, constructed from layer after layer of similar cells. At the lowest level of the epidermis there is continual cell re-growth, resulting in the layers above being forced upward until, no longer living, the cells reach the exterior and flake off. The epidermis acts as the protective barrier of the skin, its structure providing:

- photo protection (contains melanin);
- a metabolic barrier; and
- immunologic features.

The dermis lies below and is contiguous with the epidermis. The architecture of the dermis is far more complex, consisting

of an interwoven network of different fibres designed to suspend the local blood and lymphatic vessels, and to support the sweat glands and hair follicles. Also contained within the dermis are a multitude of important complex plexi of nerve endings. Their function is to ensure that constant communication is maintained, via the skin, between the exterior and the appropriate internal body systems. It is via the complex neuro anatomy of the skin that the masseur, through the medium of touch, communicates and influences the body mass.

MUSCULAR SYSTEM

Body massage is primarily involved with skeletal muscle, responsible for movement. Smooth or visceral muscle, as the name suggests, is concerned with the control and movement of internal organs or viscera. Cardiac muscle is a combination of skeletal and smooth muscle – the specialist structure of the heart enjoying its own blood supply, the coronary supply and also an independent nerve supply.

Certain acu points are claimed to influence the behaviour of both viscera and the heart. It is therefore essential than an accurate history be supplied by a person or by a horse's vet if either require specialist massage, no matter which technique is chosen. There are a number of recorded cases or persons who have suffered heart arrest following inappropriate point stimulation by untutored persons. Colic in the horse is a veterinary problem, not a massage problem.

Muscles are a living tissue, maintained in a constant state of readiness for action in both man and horse – they are also required to maintain an appropriate posture against the forces of gravity. Muscles need to have fuel, temperature regulation, oxygen, and waste removal. Their structures are continually remodelling and rebuilding, either in response to an increased workload or following normal activity. All muscles span at least one joint, they are described anatomically as having an origin and an insertion. The origin or source of a muscle is sited at an area nearer the body centre, the insertion is distal to the body centre.

The movement muscles are composed of

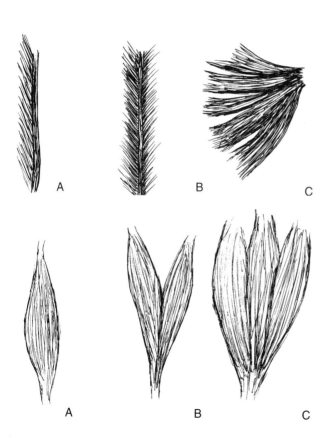

Fibre arrangement for support.
A pennate
B bipennate
C serrated

Fibre arrangement for motion.
A strap
B biceptal
C triceptal
Biceptal muscle has two origins and one insertion. Triceptal muscle has three origins and one insertion.

40

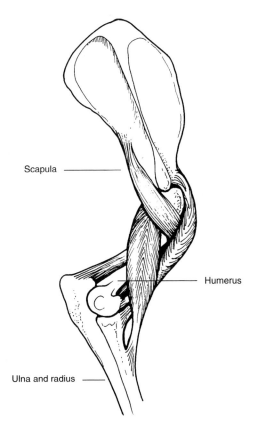

Scapula

Humerus

Ulna and radius

Deep muscles winding around the shoulder joint – lateral aspect, right shoulder.

a pattern of long, highly elastic fibres. Some possess several origins, their terminal fibres interweaving to form a single tendinous insertion. This arrangement produces the power required not only to move long levers but also to sustain the lever in the appropriate position during weight transference.

The postural muscles, which support the skeleton, differ in their fibre arrangement from those involved in movement. The muscles closest to the skeleton have short fibres to produce strength, and some literally wind around joints to provide support.

Some muscles require a greater area of attachment than can comfortably be offered by the bones of the skeleton alone, so areas of tissue known as fascia are present within skeletal muscle arrangements. These areas allow muscle fibres to 'marry' into the fibre construction of the fascia, increasing the area available for muscle anchorage. This type of fascia should not be confused with connective tissue fascia, whose function when associated with muscle tissue is to envelope each individual muscle, thus providing constraint and ensuring that power is not dissipated during muscle activity. As the outer fascial sheath ensures the individual muscle mass is contained, rather than being able to spread in any direction during contraction. The arrangement also keeps each muscle in its correct place, connecting loosely with adjacent muscle or adjoining local structure. Connective tissue fascia also serves as a support medium for blood vessels and nerves.

The human body mass will allow for the manipulation of deep muscle. When sitting in a relaxed situation with the back, neck and head fully supported, there will be little or no postural muscle activity; if recumbant and all muscles should be relaxed. The masseur will then be able to move or manipulate muscle tissue, which will influence the removal or reduction of some types of blood-borne metabolic waste. Secondary muscle relaxation can occur following toxic removal/reduction.

In the horse, due to the extent of the muscle masses and the fact that the animal is standing, resisting gravity by muscle activity, the deep-sited muscles are probably only influenced as the result of a secondary effect associated with superficial influence.

DIGESTIVE SYSTEM

The digestive system provides the fuel for activity, the components required for repair and maintenance of the body, and deals with the disposal of solid waste.

CARDIO-VASCULAR SYSTEM

The tubular vessels of the cardio-vascular system, namely the arterial vessels, capillaries and veins, infiltrate the entire body mass.

Arterial Vessels

Arterial vessels provide, via the circulating blood, a means of transportation for essential gases and nutrients. The pressure to ensure blood flow throughout the arterial system, provided by the pumping mechanism of the heart, necessitates that arteries are constructed with thick, dense, muscular walls to withstand 'blood pressure'.

Massage does not affect arterial blood flow. The circulating arterial blood passes from the arterial complex into the capillary network.

Capillaries

The microscopically thin walls of these minute vessels are constructed from complex single cells. Within the capillary complex, which might be imagined as a multi-dimensional spider's web, blood pressure reduces to allow blood-borne components to migrate outward into the tissues in response to cell and chemical command.

Waste diffuses inwards to travel, via the network existing between capillaries and

veins, through the venous part of the circulatory system, which provides transportation to the recycling or waste disposal units of the body.

Veins

Blood is under minimal internal pressure in the veins and so thick, pressure-resistant walls are not required. Compression and relaxation plays a major part in maintaining venous blood flow. Working muscle provides this requirement, although pressure forces vary according to the muscle activity. To avoid back flow, veins contain non-return valves.

It is assumed that pressure followed by release, the basis of the Swedish massage compressive techniques known as petrissage, achieves a similar effect to that of working muscle by influencing venous vessels lying within the tissues of the masseur's target area.

RESPIRATORY SYSTEM

The source of oxygen from inhaled air, also a means of waste removal (carbon dioxide) and heat loss.

LYMPHATIC SYSTEM

The function of the lymphatic or immune system is to fight invasion by disease-bearing organisms. The lymphatic vessels run, for the most part, in areas where the system exists, in parallel with the vessels of the venous system.

Massage influences the flow of lymph when the fluid is contained within the vessels of the system, but is ineffective if the fluid has migrated to the intra-cellular spaces. It is contra-indicated in the presence of known infection, lest the disease is spread from the primary site to other areas.

RENAL SYSTEM

The function of the renal system is to recycle liquids and dispose of liquid waste in the urine.

NERVOUS SYSTEM

The nervous system is responsible for communication between every body system and controlling every body function from metabolism to movement. Millions of nerve impulses are continuously reaching the brain from the body's sense receptors, and incalculable numbers are leaving the brain with instructions for the movement of muscles, joints, bones, tendons and liga-ments, together with instructions for organs and systems.

If we could unravel a nerve, the main axon or trunk would resemble the construction of a piece of string. To form a nerve, specialist cells are joined in a linear fashion forming thread-like filaments which, when packed together, form a line for communication between structure and command post. Each axon terminates at or leaves from a nerve cell. The shape of the nerve cells vary according to their specific recording and transmitting abili-ties and each type is individually named. All possess tiny, branching terminal fila-ments called dendrites. It is via these structures that messages are both trans-mitted and received.

Receptors of the nervous system record all the signals received from the hands of the masseur. These signals are not received directly – they must first be transmitted through the medium of the largest of the body systems, the skin. The signals are recorded, their content examined, the effects required deduced and the appropriate commands trans-mitted to the target area.

Even with the advancements afforded by modern scientific research, the com-plexity of the system is such that it remains imperfectly understood, and further description of its functions is not pertinent to this text. However, as it is from these reactive responses that the body responses to touch techniques must result, some basic understanding of the nervous system is required.

Central Nervous System (CNS)

This section of the nervous system, composed of the brain housed in the skull, and its extension, the spinal cord, con-tained within a bone canal formed by the vertebrae, could be described as the body's computer.

Peripheral Nervous System (PNS)

The nerves of the PNS link every part of the body to the CNS. Other than the twelve pairs of cranial nerves, which pass direct from the brain into the body mass through apertures in the skull, the nerves of the PNS are sourced from the spinal cord. The nerves leave the cord in pairs at each intra-vertebral space, one nerve from each side of the cord, to emerge into the body mass through small bone channels formed by the shapes of the vertebral bodies. Each nerve originates from two spinal roots, which merge immediately after leaving the spinal cord to form a single mixed nerve known as a lower motor neurone.

The motor nerve fibres are those arising from the anterior root. Their function is to transmit commands originating in the brain and passed down the spinal cord. When collected, these commands are delivered to the targeted area of the body mass. The sensory nerve fibres arise from the posterior root: their function is to transmit messages back to the spinal cord and thence to the brain.

These main nerves divide and join branches from other PNS nerves to create complex plexi. The nerves divide and subdivide, each final filament terminating in a specialist cell. A stimulus will trigger a chemical release by the cell which will lead to a programmed reaction. The functions attributed to these nerves, now known as peripheral nerves, might be compared to computer software programs.

Nerve endings (neural receptors) are very complex, each type possessing a design specific to a particular function. All nerve endings are activated by a series of complex, programmed, chemical reactions that occur in response to a wide variety of stimuli. Nerve endings influenced during massage and allied therapies are those concerned with touch, pressure, stretching, temperature, and passive movement.

Touch Receptors

Effleurage   Stimulates a natural opiate release, reducing the sensation of pain and promoting general relaxation.

Tapotment   Produces a stimulatory effect by increasing local circulatory activity and so 'warming' targeted tissues. Continuous, repetitive, rhythmic stimuli evoke the 'gate response', a naturally present pain-relieving mechanism described by Melzak and Wall in *The Gate Theory of Pain* (*see* Bibliography).

TTEAM   The localized sites selected for the application of the techniques of TTEAM produce relaxation in areas of the body where tension is creating secondary pain. The stimulatory procedures also enhance body awareness. Specialized techniques based on voice direction methods and exercises used to re-balance movement patterns in human patients have been adapted for use with a horse.

Pressure Receptors

Acupressure   By using carefully selected points, acupressure will re-balance body energy following disruption of normal energy flow.

Trigger point stimulation   Trigger points appear to be located in identical sites to those used in acupressure and react in a similar manner.

Petrissage   Influences the movement of venous blood and lymph.

Stretch Receptors

Bowen Technique	Influences energy balance via the subcutaneous mech-anoreceptors of the ANS.
CTM	Influences energy balance via the mechanoreceptors sited in connective tissue of the ANS.
Passive stretching	Affects tissue via stretch receptors sited in all soft tissue structures.

Thermal Receptors

Cryo-therapy	Lowers the superficial tissue temperature, causing local vasoconstriction and reducing local metabolic activity.
Heat	Raises the superficial tissue temperature causing local vasodilation.

Joint pro-prioceptors	Passive movements establish and maintain intercommunication between joints, ligaments, supporting muscles and tendon structures following injury.

Autonomic Nervous System (ANS)

This section of the nervous system controls and is responsible for all auto-matic bodily functions – digestion, respiration, temperature control, saliva-tion – to name but a few. ANS may be divided into two groups – sympathetic and parasympathetic. There is continual interplay between the reflex actions of both sympathetic and parasympathetic fibres in order to achieve the required state of balance.

5 Comparative and Surface Anatomy —

It is important for the masseur to be able to read the 'body map' – anatomical markers are an essential guide both for general massage and when using acupressure. The location of all acu points are described in the original Chinese texts and can be identified by locating the described anatomical point and, using very precise measurements, moving to the acu point.

While the nervous systems of man and the horse are considered by most to have the same features, this assumption is incorrect. The pyramidal tract is a notable example. This tract, which is involved in the manipulative skills of the digits, is well developed in man. The horse, being devoid of multiple fingers and toes, does not require a communicating tract. Therefore it is no surprise that the tract barely exists in the spinal cord of the horse.

Consider also that at birth the horse possesses a fully developed nervous system, allowing the new-born foal to run with its dam within a few minutes of birth, recognize its mother amongst a herd, communicate – in fact behave exactly as an adult animal. In comparison, the human is totally helpless at birth, taking months to learn to stand, communicate, recognize and visualize.

It is important to remember that because man and the horse have different neurological responses, the response to a treatment may also vary.

COMPARATIVE ANATOMY

Cervical Vertebrae

Both species have seven cervical vertebrae and seven pairs of cervical nerves.

Shoulder Blades

Both species have a pair of shoulder blades (scapulae). In the horse, the spines lie at an angle across the chest wall; in man, they lie parallel to the ground when in the standing position. The lie of the scapular spine in the horse determines the stride length, a vertical spine results in a short stride, a 'laid back' spine allows a longer stride. (Massage cannot influence this, it is a fact of conformation.)

Collar Bone

The horse has no collar bones (clavicle). Man has a pair, which increase the strength of his shoulder complex.

Ribs

Man has twelve pairs of ribs and thoracic nerves, the horse has eighteen.

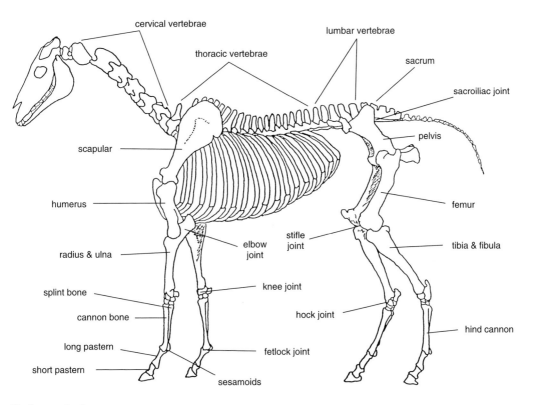

Skeleton of a horse.

Lumbar Vertebrae

Man has five lumbar vertebrae; the horse generally has six, sometimes seven, and usually five in the Arabian. Consequently, man has five pairs of lumbar nerves and the horse may have five, six or seven pairs.

Sacrum

This is fused in both species.

Tail Bone

The tail bone (coccyx) is longer in the horse than in man.

Back

From the base of the skull to the pelvis, the human back should be stable at the junction between the last lumbar vertebrae and the pelvis, L5/S1, and at junction of neck to chest C7/T1. In the horse these segments enjoy the greatest amount of mobility in the equine back.

Skeleton

The human skeleton, mass for mass, is greater than that of the horse, whose skeleton is remarkably light when its muscle mass is considered. It follows that the muscle mass of the horse requires

47

The human skeleton.

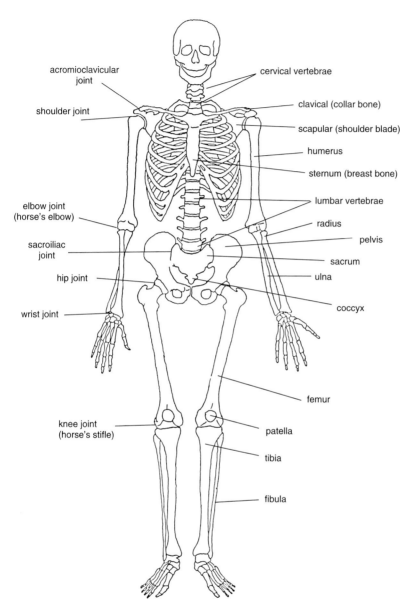

acromioclavicular joint

cervical vertebrae

shoulder joint

clavical (collar bone)

scapular (shoulder blade)

humerus

sternum (breast bone)

elbow joint (horse's elbow)

lumbar vertebrae

radius

sacroiliac joint

pelvis

sacrum

hip joint

ulna

wrist joint

coccyx

femur

knee joint (horse's stifle)

patella

tibia

fibula

considerably more pressure during the administration of certain of the Swedish massage techniques, than does the muscle mass of man.

Both species possess deep muscles whose function is to ensure a stable basic frame. This frame, known as the axial skeleton, enables the appendicular skeleton, when converted to levers by their musculature, to move the main frame as a whole.

A Facial crest
B Temporal line
C Angle of lower jaw
D Parotid gland
E Poll and reflex
    point area
F Wings of the Atlas
G Cervical vertebrae
H Tip of sternum
I   Point of shoulder
J   Spine of the scapula
K Point of the elbow,
    ulna
L Accessory carpal
    bone
M Lateral sesamoid
N Posterior superior
    spines
O Jumpers bumps,
    tuber sacrale
P Point of hip, tuber
    coccae
Q Greater trochanter
R Stifle joint
S Hock

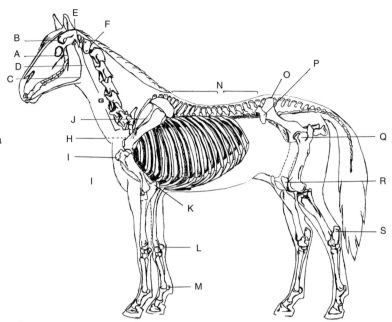

SURFACE ANATOMY OF THE HORSE

It is essential that every aspiring masseur should have an appreciation of equine surface anatomy. It is not possible to appreciate movement sequences and to locate both the directional lie and shape of the muscle groups responsible for them, unless the shape of the skeleton and location of the limbs upon the axial frame are clearly understood.

A familiarity with the sensation of the texture of bone is also very important, otherwise it may be mistaken for muscle spasm. The best way to learn surface anatomy is to feel the entire body surface with your hands, preferably with your eyes closed. For safety reasons, a companion to hold the horse is advisable.

Head

Start by feeling the head. There is very little muscle covering this area other than the cheek (masseter) muscle. The facial crest lies just in front of the cheek muscle and behind the eye. Above the eye is the frontal bone, the upper rim is called the temporal line. Trace the angle of the jawbones.

Glands

A soft area, sometimes felt just as the jawbone angles upward and forward, is created by glands: the lowest is the mandibular gland, slightly above is the parotid gland.

Work upward to the poll – this area needs a careful light touch, as, just behind

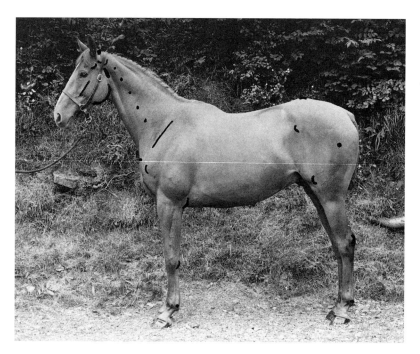

Superficial bone landmarks. These correspond to those shown on the picture on page 49.

the ears, two highly volatile reflex points are sited. In the wild, the natural predators of the horse are the big cat family. If a cat tries to break the horse's neck at the poll, the horse automatically responds by shaking the head violently. Do not be surprised if the horse reacts with a violent unanticipated head shake, or sudden upward head movement in response to pressure from your fingers. You have learnt an area to be approached with caution in the future.

Neck

The bones of the neck lie low, just above the horse's airway (trachea), not, as is commonly assumed, just under the mane.

There are seven cervical vertebrae. The first, the axis, forms the poll; the wings of the second bone, the atlas, are visible and easily felt below and behind the ears. The sides of the next four bones, C3, C4, C5, and sometimes C6 can be identified, but the seventh lies too deep, placed centrally between the shoulders and joining the neck to the barrel-like thoracic, or rib, cage.

Chest and Shoulders

Feel the front of the chest (thorax). Centrally, at the base of the neck, the tip of the sternum (wishbone) is easy to feel. On either side are two clearly defined areas of muscle. Moving the hands outward, bone can be felt in the area just above the junction of the front leg to the body – this area is known as the point of the shoulder. The bone is the upper end of the humerus, palpable as it

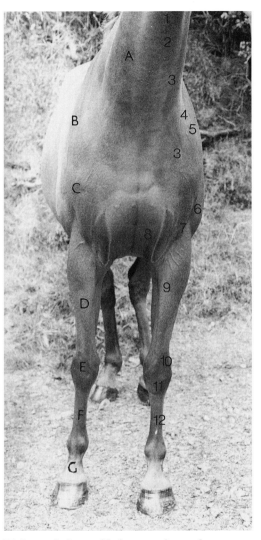

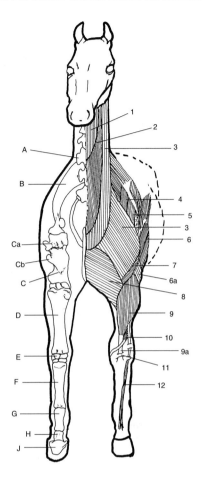

Right and above: *Skeleton and muscles, anterior aspect.*

Skeleton	Muscles
A Cervical vertebrae	1 Sternothyrohyoid
B Scapula (shoulder blade)	2 Sternocephalic
	3 Brachiocephalic
C Humerus (a) point of shoulder	4 Deep pectoral
	5 Supraspinatus
D Radius	6/6a Long and lateral head of triceps
E Carpal (knee joint)	
F Cannon bone	7 Brachialis
G Long pastern, (1st phalanx)	8 Superficial pectoral
	9 Extensor carpi radialis
H Short pastern, (2nd phalanx)	10 Extensor carpi obliquus
J Pedal bone (3rd phalanx)	11 Annular ligaments
	12 Common digital extensor tendon

lies just below the skin. The actual shoulder joint lies deep in this area and cannot be felt.

The next major landmark is the ridge of bone running as a distinct line from just below the wither area downward and forward towards the point of the shoulder. This ridge is formed by the spine of the

51

shoulder blade, the bone known as the scapular.

Located at the top and to the back of the front leg, the point of the elbow is easy to feel formed by the tip of the bone called the ulna, this point lies at the outer side of the armpit (axilla), which is very important to all masseurs, for venous blood from the head, neck, forelimbs, shoulders and front part of the chest return to this area via large, specialist veins. After being cleansed of waste, the blood returns to the arterial delivery system to be reloaded with nutrients. All massage strokes performed over the front (cranial) aspect of the horse should be directed towards the armpit.

Forelimb

All the structures of the forelimb (thoracic limb) are easily identified and located.

The accessory knee (carpal) bone lying as a protuberance at the back of the knee

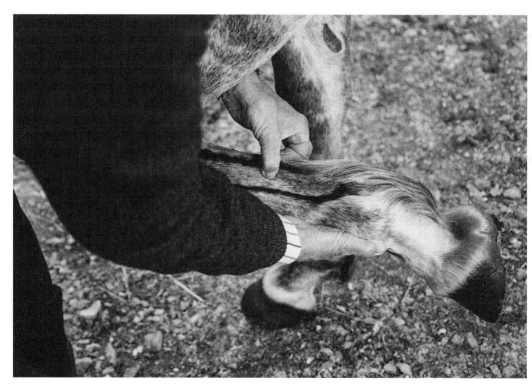

The superficial flexor tendon is held between finger and thumb, this hold also influences the deep flexor tendon, as the superficial wraps around the deep in a U-shaped fashion. The suspensory ligament lies immediately adjacent to the palmar surface of the cannon bone, dividing into two branches just above the fetlock joint. The sesamoid bones are contained one within each branch, one medially, one laterally sited. The branches then angle forward to be inserted on the dorsal aspect.

is easy to feel. The structures lying behind the cannon bone are best felt with the horse's foot off the ground and the knee flexed. It is then possible to identify the superficial digital flexor tendon, the deep digital flexor tendon, the suspensory ligament, the inferior check ligament and the medial and lateral sesamoid bones.

In a healthy foot the coronet band should feel soft, lying either parallel to the hoof wall, or feeling slightly concave. A bulging, convex coronet, is often synonymous with foot discomfort.

Ribcage and Back

The ribcage is easily identified, but the underside of the cage, and backward towards the sheath/teats area should not be palpated. This area, just like the poll, contains a mass of reflex sensors, all concerned with survival. It is a reflex response, not malice, which causes the horse to kick if any of these points are inadvertently stimulated.

Certain acupressure/puncture points are located in the belly. However, only

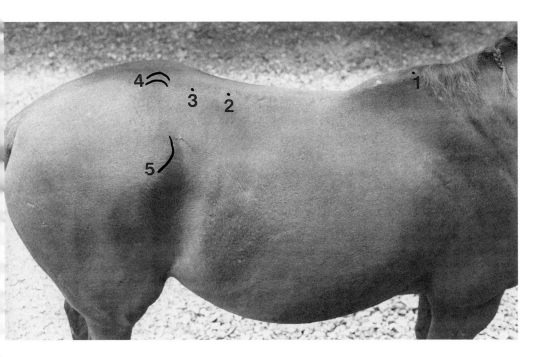

The equine back.

1   *The tip of the posterior superior spine of the 3rd thoracic vertebrae, T3.*
2   *Tip of the posterior superior spine of the 18th thoracic vertebrae, T18.*
3   *Tip of the posterior superior spine of the 5th lumbar vertebrae, L5. The posterior superior spine of L6 cannot be palpated, it lies deep below the two ilial wings where, at its junction with the 1st sacral body, the two bones, L6 S1, form the most important hinge of the equine back, the lumbo sacral joint.*
4   *Jumpers bumps. Tuber sacrale.*
5   *Point of hip. Tuber coccae.*

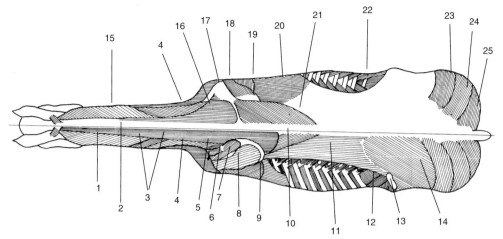

The neck and back from above.

Deep muscles
1 Splenius.
2 Rhomboid.
3 Serratus ventralis (cervical fibres).
4 Brachiocephalic.
5 Deep pectoral (cranial fibres).
6 Serratus ventralis.
7 Spine of scapular.
8 Infraspinatus.
9 Triceps.
10 Part of longissimus.
11 Longissimus.
12 Transverse abdominal.
13 Internal abdominal oblique.
14 Medial gluteal.

Superficial muscles
15 Splenius cervicis.
 4 Brachiocephalic.
16 Trapezius.
17 Spine of scapular.
18 Deltoid.
19 Triceps.
20 Latissimus dorsi.
21 Trapezius.
22 External abdominal oblique.
23 Superficial gluteal.
24 Biceps femoris.
25 Semitendinosus.

careful measurement to determine location will ensure a positive, rather than an adverse reaction.

The tips of the long bone spines running from the vertebral bodies upward to the centre of the back, beginning with that of the third thoracic vertebrae, found just in front of the withers, can be felt with the fingers. These tips are not bone, but a specialist cartilage affording attachment for a supporting ligament of the back – the posterior superior spinous ligament. They palpate differently to true bone.

Where the loins join the hindquarters, there should be a sudden dip. This is normal, not, as is sometimes suggested, because the horse has a bad back. The next palpable landmarks are the two 'jumper's bumps', the tuber sacrale (*see* photograph on p.53).

Pelvis

Moving outward from the tuber sacrale, the huge bulk of the hindquarter muscles stretch to the point of the hip (tuber

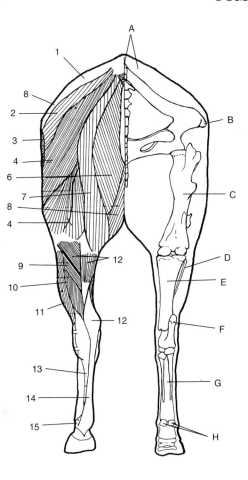

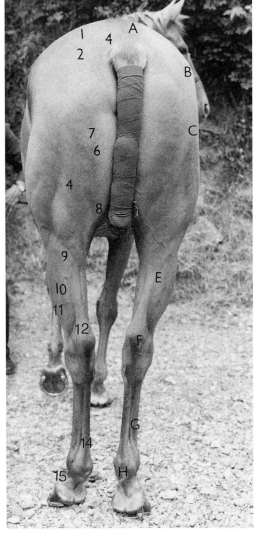

Above and right: *The muscles and skeleton viewed from behind.*

Muscles
1 *Gluteal fascia.*
2 *Superficial gluteal.*
3 *Tensor fascial muscle.*
4 *Biceps femoris.*
6 *Semitendinosus*
7 *Semimembranosus*
8 *Gracilis.*
9 *Soleus.*
10 *Flexor digitorum profundis.*
11 *Extensor digitorum lateralis.*
12 *Gastrocnemius.*
13 *Deep flexor tendon.*
14 *Superficial flexor tendon.*
15 *Lateral branch suspensory.*

Skeleton
A *Tuber sacrale (jumpers bumps).*
B *Tuber coxae (point of hip).*
C *Femur.*
D *fibula.*
E *Tibia and fused fibula*
F *Point of hock.*
G *Cannon and splints.*
H *Sesamoid bones, medial and lateral.*

55

coccae), a cartilage-covered bone prominence. Lying at the outermost point of the ilium, itself a wing of bone forming the upper brim of the pelvis, the points of the hip have nothing to do with the hip joint.

The hip joint is not palpable, lying too deep below the overlying muscles. A bone point, a part of the thigh bone (femur) can be located on fit horses. Known as the greater trochanter, this bone point is a useful landmark for masseurs.

Just as the armpits in the front of the horse are important for the returning venous blood, so the groin area is important as a collection point at the rear (caudal) end of the horse. The groin lies deep to the greater trochanter, inside the hind leg and backward from the stifle joint, the next palpable landmark. Because of the groin's importance as a collection point, massage strokes should be directed towards the groin when working over the loins and hind limbs of the horse. However, like humans, horses do not appreciate massage in the groin area itself.

Hind Limb

The hind limbs of the horse are slightly longer than the forelimbs. The hock is easily recognized and palpated. The structures below the hock joint mirror those of the forelimbs.

ANATOMY OF MOVEMENT OF THE HORSE

The horse has evolved in a manner that has provided the animal with an economic, high speed, locomotor function ability, which has ensured the survival of the species

in the face of danger from predators.

By domesticating the horse, man has harnessed some these abilities but also persuaded it to perform unnatural movement sequences. Domesticity has not, however, changed the fundamental characteristics of the original wild horse, and many of the problems to which the animal is subject in captivity are as a result of man's interference.

Movement is produced by muscular activity, necessitating both neuromuscular co-ordination and adequate fuel. As in every situation when energy is expended, waste is a secondary factor. In a natural situation, the horse cleanses its muscles of accumulated waste by walking long distances after periods of activity. Due to the confines imposed by stabling, the horse is unable to cleanse its systems as it would under natural conditions.

The horse is a herbivore designed to eat off the ground, with a digestive system required to ingest large quantities of green, succulent bulk containing a high proportion of fluid. Man stables the horse, feeds it from a manger rather than allowing it to eat off the ground, which disturbs its digestive processes, and offers a proprietary 'mix' or nuts, with dry bulk in the form of hay.

Masseurs should be aware that no massage technique or allied therapy can ensure the horse will remain in good health, if the factors which created the problem still exist.

MOVEMENT OF THE APPENDICULAR SKELETON

The horse moves by using muscles to convert the bones forming its limbs to a

The thoracic and pelvic levers.

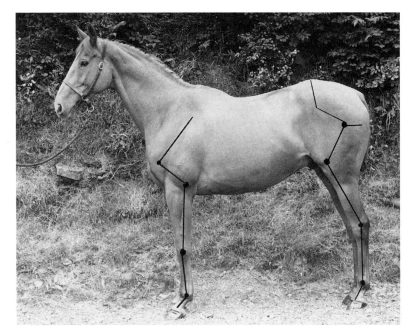

Bones of the appendicular skeleton, which form the thoracic and pelvic levers.

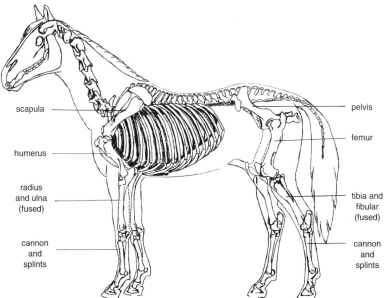

scapula

humerus

radius
and ulna
(fused)

cannon
and
splints

pelvis

femur

tibia and
fibular
(fused)

cannon
and
splints

system of variable, functionally angled levers. The angularity and length of the levers change during motion in a repetitive sequence, resulting in efficient, economic movement.

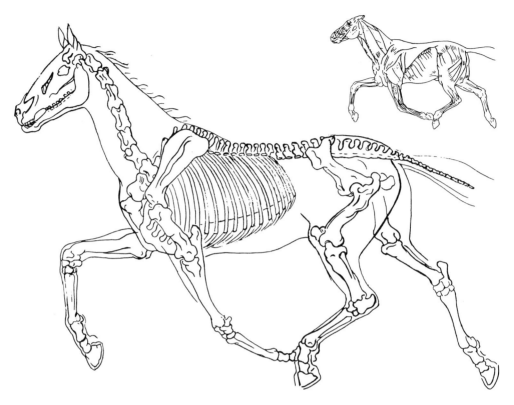

The limbs are formed into a series of variable levers by the muscles to produce movement.

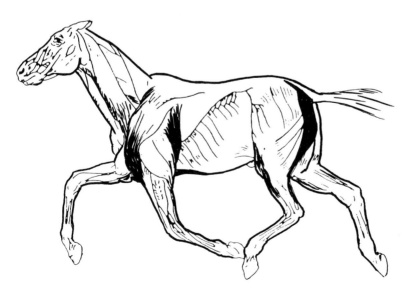

Muscles create levers and by moving the levers produce motion.

Forelimb

Bones Involved in Movement of the
Forelimb are the:

- scapula (shoulder bone);
- humerus (upper arm);
- radius and ulna fused as one (lower arm); and
- cannon, splint, sesamoid and pastern bones.

Joints Involved in Movement of the
Forelimb are:

- The shoulder joint, formed between the shallow cup at the distal end of the scapula and the rounded, half-spherical head of the humerus. The construction allows multi-axial movement.
- The elbow joint, formed between the distal end of the humerus and the proximal end of the fused radius and ulna. The construction forms a hinge joint.
- The knee (carpal) joint. This is formed from a number of bones. In the centre, two rows of small bones are arranged one above the other. The distal end of the radius moves against the upper aspect of the top row. The platform created by the top of the cannon and the two splint bones moves against the lower surface of the lower row. The joint is primarily designed as a hinge, but tendon arrangement in some horses produces a rotation, creating a dishing action.
- The fetlock and pastern joints are hinge joints that rely on weight forces and elastic recoil for activity, not muscle action.

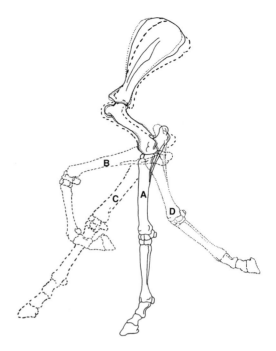

Anatomy of movement – forelimb.

A   *normal stance*   B   *first stage of advancement*
C   *straightening limb* D   *retracting limb.*

Movement of the Forelimb
There is no true joint between the forelimb and the body mass, the limb is literally hung from the withers. The muscle arrangement produces a pendulum-type action of the shoulder bone during limb activity. Stability is maintained by the subscapularis, which holds the scapula to the chest wall. This muscle cannot be massaged – it is covered in its entirety by the scapula.

The scapula, the first bone comprising the forelimb, is also attached to the withers by the fan-like trapezius muscle. The widest part of the fan extends from mid-neck to well behind the withers. The narrowest part of the fan is attached to the upper (dorsal) border of the scapula. Contraction of the cranial fibres of the trapezius, assist in rotating the scapula forward, changing the angle of the shoulder joint to allow, by appropriate muscle recruitment, extension at the joint enabling the horse to move the forelimb forward from the body mass. (*See* the diagram on page 59.) This action represents a forward swing of the pendulum.

The muscles controlling the forelimb must lift the forearm and maintain momentary suspension as the shoulder bone angles to position the shoulder joint. Then, from the elbow the muscles must both straighten and lower the limb to place the foot on the ground, maintaining stability of the limb as the body weight passes over the planted forefoot. After the body weight passes beyond the vertical of the supporting forelimb, and the limb is positioned beneath the mid-body, a hind limb supplies temporary balance through ground contact.

At this stage, the forelimb is lifted and flexed. To align the shoulder joint for flexion, the caudal fibres of trapezius lying behind the shoulder bone contract. This action represents a backward swing of the pendulum.

Energy created by overstretch and loaded in the tendons of the lower limb, snap the foot and fetlock to their normal position; then the limb is carried forward in a flexed position from under the body mass for the cycle to be repeated.

Hind Limb

Bones Involved in Movement of the Hind (Pelvic) Limb are the:

- pelvis;
- femur (thigh bone);
- second thigh or gaskin (tibia and fibula, fused); and
- cannon, splint, sesamoid and pastern bones.

Joints Involved in Movement of the Hind Limb are:

- The hip joint. Formed by a deep saucer or acetabulum sited on the pelvis. The rounded femoral head is constructed with an internal ligament running between socket and head. The construction allows multi-axial movement. The internal ligament adds strength.
- The stifle joint. Formed by the distal end of the femur and proximal end of the fused tibia and fibula, the stifle joint is constructed with two internal ligaments – the cruciate ligaments, and two cartilages – the menisci. The patella (kneecap), encased within the tendon of the quadriceps, forms part of the front of the joint. The construction is that of a hinge joint. The internal ligaments and patella add strength and stability.
- The hock joint. Formed from a number of bones. Movement takes place between the distal end of the fused tibia and fibula and the calcaneum, the largest of the bones forming the joint. Below the calcaneum, two rows of small bones form the middle of the joint – the lower aspect of the distal row attached to the platform formed by the proximal end of the cannon and splint bones. The construction forms a hinge joint.
- The fetlock and pastern joints. These are all hinge joints and rely on weight forces and elastic recoil for movement, not muscle activity.

Movement of the Hind Limb

The muscles of the hind limb flex the hip, stifle and hock; carry the limb under the body in a flexed position; then lower the limb to plant the foot. As the foot meets the ground, muscles both stabilize and straighten the limb, producing an immense power thrust to drive the entire body mass forward over the planted forelimb. After the limb has completed full thrust it is lifted, the foot and fetlock snap into position, and the limb is brought under the body for the cycle to be repeated.

Dependent upon the gait adopted, the number of limbs in contact with the ground at any one time varies, as does the contact sequence. At fast paces and while jumping, there are periods of total suspension with no ground contact. In such situations, despite economic energy usage, the stresses to the structures of the leading forelimb increase dramatically due to the stretch and recoil facility of the tendons, whose action literally springs the horse off the ground.

The lateral movements required in dressage necessitate active interplay between muscles whose normal role is to stabilize limbs rather than move them, preventing them falling inward (adduction) or outward (abduction). In order to work effectively on muscles put under unnatural stress, all masseurs should study gait and be familiar with competition requirements. They should also be familiar with conformation in order to appreciate the limitations it may impose on gait ability. For example, a horse with a very straight hind leg will have difficulty engaging its hocks to perform some dressage movements. Similarly, a horse with a very straight shoulder will not be able to achieve a fore-

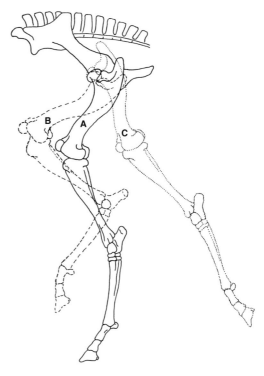

Anatomy of movement – hind limb.

A   *normal stance*
B   *first stage prior to thrust*
C   *thrust.*

limb extension stride to match that of a horse with a laid-back shoulder. Massage cannot alter these factors, but it will help to relieve the muscle discomfort created in limbs and body after a horse has been asked, as is often the case, to perform movements of which, due to conformation, it is incapable.

MOVEMENT OF THE AXIAL SKELETON

Compared to the appendicular skeleton, the range of movement of the joints throughout the axial skeleton is very restricted.

Bones of the Axial Skeleton

- Cervical vertebrae – seven;
- thoracic vertebrae – eighteen;
- ribs – eighteen pairs;
- sternum;
- lumbar vertebrae – six, in a long-backed horse – seven, in the Arabian – usually five;
- sacrum – five fused bones;
- tail bones (coccageal vertebrae) – between eighteen and twenty-one; and
- pelvic bones.

The thoracic vertebrae together with the ribs and sternum form the thoracic cage. The pelvic bones together with the sacrum form a cave-like ring of bone to which the femur is attached by an inter-articular ligament at the hip joint.

Joints of the Axial Skeleton

Intervertebral joints exist between the bodies of all the vertebrae from C1 to the junction of L6 and S1. With the exception of the first and second cervical joints, all possess intervertebral discs. These discs are of a differing construction to those of man. Accounting for a quarter of the total length of the backbone, they are formed from a dense fibrous matrix. The design allows for strength and shock absorption, but minimal movement.

Three areas enjoy a reasonable movement range. In the neck, most movement occurs at its base, the junction between the last neck vertebrae C7, and the first of the chest T1.

At the lumbar sacral junction L6 S1, a joint formed between the last lumbar vertebrae and the first sacral allows local flexion as the hind limb moves under the body, followed by extension as the hind limb thrusts the body mass forward. The third area is the junction between the last thoracic vertebrae T18, and the first lumbar vertebrae L1, where a very small range of flexion and extension is present.

The action of the ribs is similar to that of a bucket handle, a minute amount of rotation occurring both at the junction of each rib to its parent thoracic vertebrae, and in the case of the first ten pairs of ribs with the sternum.

The design of the thoracic cage can be visualized as an upturned, flat-bottomed rowing boat, the ribs represented by the ribs of the craft, the narrow prow as the chest, the structure widening towards the stern.

The neck could be likened to the jib arm of a crane, projecting well forward of the body mass, the heavy head acting as a counterbalance weight. Neck position and function is important, not only to assist balance but also to ensure through traction forces, created by the nuchal ligament and disseminated throughout the back, as the ligament continues as the supra spinous ligament, that the back remains stable. Movement is minimized during activity, other than at the lumbar sacral junction.

The back, from withers to loins, remains remarkably stable during any activity, the musculature being designed for support rather than activity.

MUSCLES

The majority of books treat muscles in much the same way as anatomical texts

- each muscle is named and individually described. However, looking at the diagrams or anatomical drawings can make it difficult to appreciate that in the living body, muscles are not single entities.

Muscles are arranged as groups and, with only a few exceptions, they work in groups, marry into one another, wrap around each other, and share common fascial origins and insertions. Those working as partners usually enjoy a common nerve supply. Muscle groups involved in initiating and controlling movements must work in unison – as one group contracts, the opposing group relaxes. If joints and body areas require stabilizing during movement, appropriate muscle groups are activated. This complex interaction is called co-ordination.

The masseur is working over muscle masses and should consider the groups involved in movement patterns, rather than individual muscles. The type of activity undertaken is also of importance, for the manner in which the muscles function and the range of muscle action determine both stress and fatigue levels. Frequently used terms include:

- Prime mover/agonist: initiator of movement.
- Antagonist: working in opposition to prime mover.
- Fixator: creates a transient, immovable area to enhance a movement.
- Concentric: muscles shorten during function.
- Eccentric: muscles lengthen during function. A very demanding muscle activity, not to be confused with the reciprocal relaxation of antagonistic function.
- Active: continuous activity allowing contraction followed by relaxation.

The constant changes of tension enhance circulation, thus work does not create undue fatigue in conditioned muscles.
- Static: muscles maintain a working tension against a load. A very demanding muscle activity.
- Isotonic: slight, continual contractions to resist gravity.
- Isometric: tension rather than contraction. Creates fatigue if a position has to be maintained over a long period. Static, isometric muscle activity creates a build-up of lactates, leading rapidly to discomfort and muscle fatigue.

Range of Muscle Activity

Muscles at rest are usually in a state of middle-range isotonic contraction or exhibiting a mild degree of tone in preparation for instant function.

To envisage range, joint movement becomes an integral factor. Imagine the distance between the points of origin and insertion of muscle attachment constituting an imaginary 180 degree baseline.

- Outer range: the lever is long and the structures at full stretch, the working muscle moves the joint through a range from 180° to approximately 145°. Elastic recoil, the result of full stretch, assists muscle contraction. Economic function.
- Middle range: the lever is slightly bent and contraction bends the joint from 145 through 90 degrees to 45 degrees. Efficient function of both strength and motion.
- Inner range: the movement is through a decreasing angle of 45 degrees. Little motion, fatiguing.

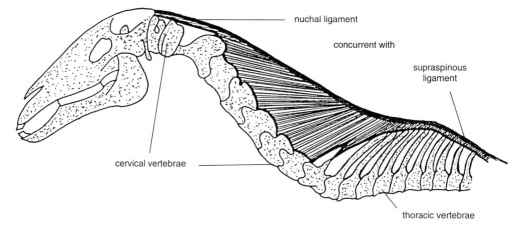

nuchal ligament

concurrent with

supraspinous ligament

cervical vertebrae

thoracic vertebrae

Nuchal ligament showing fan-like attachments to cervical vertebrae.

Group Action of Muscles

The neck is suspended from the nuchal ligament. The muscle masses are arranged between this structure and the bones of the neck in a manner that enables the horse to bend the neck from side to side, and lower and raise the head. To achieve a side bend of the neck, the muscles sited on the side to which the head turns contract, while on the other side of the neck their exact opposite relax (reciprocal relaxation).

The head needs to reach down to the ground for grazing. This action is partly muscular, but for energy conservation, the elastic properties of the nuchal ligament are involved. The structure loads with energy as the head is lowered, then the fibres employing elastic recoil assist the neck muscles to lift the head to its normal position. As in the wild, the horse will continually lower and raise the head conservation of muscle energy is essential for survival. A horse that falls on its head and as a result forces the neck sideways will injure the muscles of the side that is stretched.

A horse has to be taught, and the muscles suitably conditioned, to achieve and maintain an 'outline'. When asked to maintain this unnatural posture, often for long periods without being allowed to stretch down, off the bit, the position creates unbelievable discomfort. The neck musculature becomes fatigued and tense during both learning and schooling. Effleurage should be the first technique used to produce some relaxation, then the neck can be massaged using localized, circular techniques working the whole area between poll and withers. The expression on the horse's face will indicate areas of discomfort. To appreciate the depth of the neck musculature stand with one hand on either side of the neck and envisage the distance between your hands. This will give an idea of the pressure required to influence centrally sited tissue.

The brachiocephalic muscle runs from the poll to the front of the shoulder where the muscle fibres interlace with structures on the front of the chest. Normally working as part of the group involved in bringing the front leg forward, the muscle can change the way it works and pull the body forward over the planted

64

A *Surface contour and position of the brachio cephalic muscle. Over use creates an upside-down neck.*

B *Area where fibres of the scalene muscle can be massaged. The muscle is deep sited other than just in front of the scapular where a small section lies superficial.*

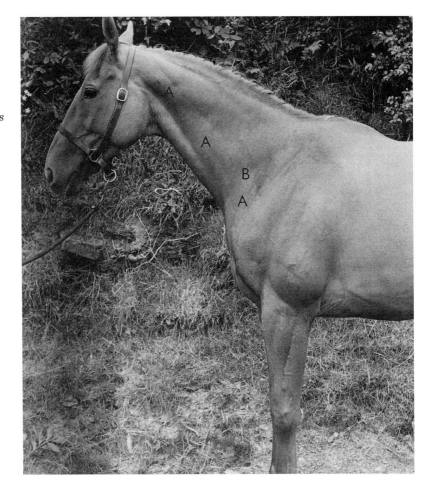

front leg. If this action is used too frequently, the muscle overdevelops and bulges in a convex curve on the under surface of the neck – this condition is described as an 'upside-down neck' and is often secondary to hind-limb or hind-quarter pain.

A group of deep neck muscles, in particular the scalene, stabilize the first rib. A stable first rib is essential for downhill work and landing after a jump. Deep massage at the base of the neck, forward of the shoulder bone at the positions of the fourth, fifth and sixth cervical

neck vertebrae where these muscles attach, will affect the group.

Forelimb and Shoulder

The muscles that advance the forelimb and stabilize the shoulder joint lie under the base of the neck over the front of the chest wall where they create a definite convexity on either side of the sternum. These muscles work with those lying on, over and in front of the scapula. These groups should be worked with all

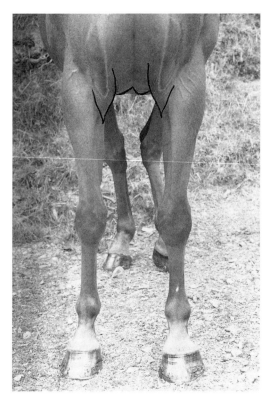

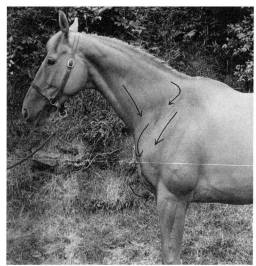

Direction of techniques for muscles involved in forelimb advancement. The groups should be worked with techniques directed down and inward towards the axilla.

The adductor muscles normally work as stabilizers but become active during lateral work in dressage.

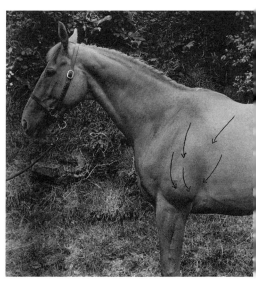

The muscles lying in, over and behind the scapula and extending to mid-ribs, retract or take the forelimb back under the body. The groups should be worked with techniques towards the axilla.

techniques directed down and inward towards the axilla.

To prevent the forelimb moving outward, away from the body mass is a group of muscles that act as adductors. Situated on the underside of the wall of the thoracic cage and lying on each side of the sternum, the muscle mass extends backward to behind the girth and down the inner side of the forelimb, to just below the chest wall. Normally working in a stabilizing role, these muscles become active in the lateral movements required in dressage. The contour formed by the group is obvious when the standing horse is viewed from the front.

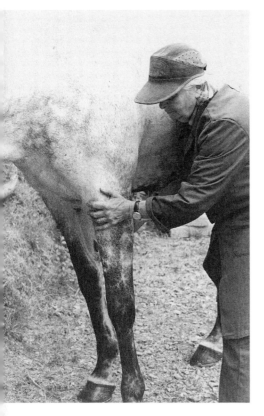 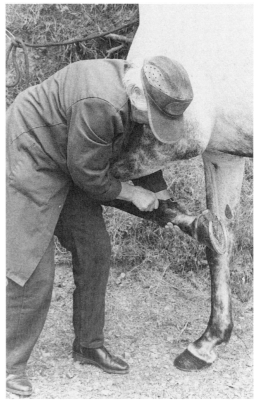

It is impossible to massage structures in tension. Due to the stay system the limbs of the horse must not relax when in a weight-bearing situation. The limb is best massaged in flexion.

With the limb in flexion, use the fingers and thumb to massage the tendons. The horse's knee rests on the masseur's thigh and the shoulder is supported by the masseur's shoulder.

The muscles lying on, over and behind the scapula, extending to the mid-ribs, take the forelimb backward.

Of particular importance is the bulky muscle group attached to the elbow: the three heads of triceps and associated fibres of serratus ventralis. Techniques should be directed down and inward toward the axilla.

The muscles of the forelimb, terminating as the lower limb tendons at the knee, lie at the back of the forearm where they can easily be palpated.

To enable the animal to remain upright, the musculature of the limbs of the standing horse must be in a state of constant tension. This makes it difficult to massage effectively – the limb is best massaged in flexion.

Due to hair lie, limb effleurage is not comfortable for the horse. Compression techniques should be used – the whole hand on the forearm, fingers or thumbs over the tendons. Coronet and frog

67

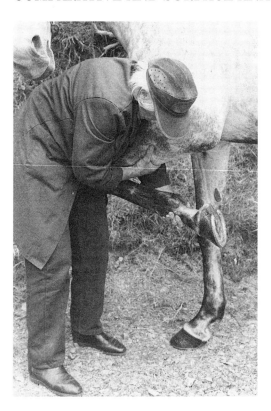

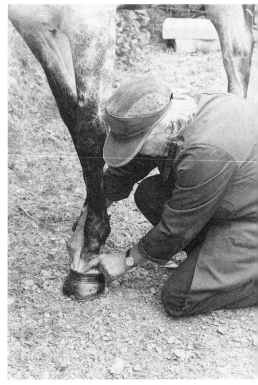

With the limb in flexion, compression techniques are used on the forearm.

Coronet and frog compression are best performed with the foot on the ground.

compression are best performed with the foot on the ground using circular, double-handed techniques, given with the thumbs or individual fingers.

Back

The back muscles, designed in a multi-pennate fibre pattern, provide support rather than movement. The muscles fill the area between the vertical spines of the bones of the back and the flat upper surface of the ribs.

Back discomfort is often caused by a poorly fitting saddle. Uneven diagonals

create a 'torque' in the loins leading to muscle discomfort in the area.

The masseur may need to stand on a box for back massage to be effective. Effleurage will usually relax the horse enough to allow the use of deeper, locally applied techniques. All techniques are bound to influence acupressure/trigger points, and zones described in the techniques of Ttouch.

Work from withers to loins. Do not massage over the ribs or abdomen. There are no active muscles over the ribs and the abdomen is not only highly sensitive but normal intestinal movement might be disturbed.

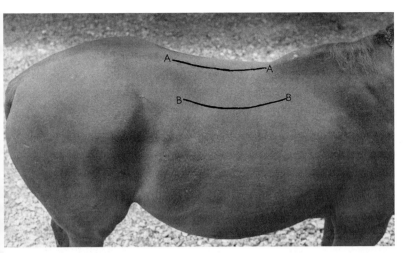

The back muscles fill the area between the vertical spines of the bones of the back, tips AA, at the flat upper surface of the ribs. The ribs begin to angle down at the line BB.

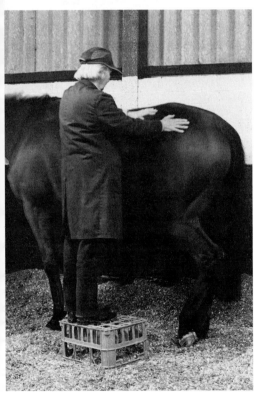

The masseur may need to stand on a box for massage to be effective.

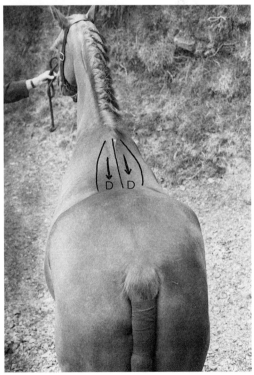

The back muscles fill the area between the vertical spines of the back and the flat upper surface of the ribs. DD shows areas of discomfort secondary to torque associated with uneven diagonals.

69

Hindquarters and Hind Limbs

Some horses appear to have very rounded quarters, others seem rather flat with very pronounced 'jumper's bump' or tuber sacrale. There are two reasons for this difference in shape. The first results from the requirements of the discipline.

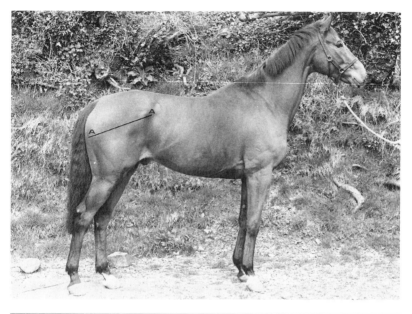

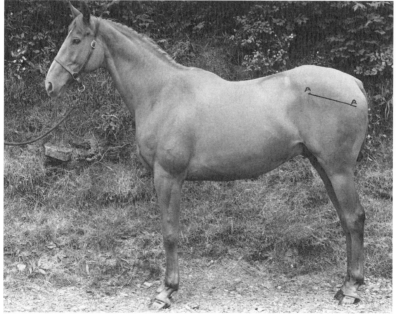

Left above and below: *The shape of the hindquarter outline varies, this may be due to muscular development secondary to discipline, or as in the case of the horses in these plates, because their conformation is disimilar. The horse above is long between the tuber coccae and tuber ischae AA, the horse below is short. The variation in the shape of the muscle mass is NOT due to weakness or muscle loss as is often supposed, but due to conformation.*

The dressage horse, working muscles in the middle range of movement will build considerable bulk, developing a different hindquarter top line to that of the flat race-horse who, working muscles in the outer range requires recoil rather than mass.

The second reason is pelvic size – the distance from the tuber coccaie (point of the hip) to the back of the pelvis tuber isichi varies the greater the distance between these two points, the flatter the muscle contour. The shorter the distance, the rounder the contour.

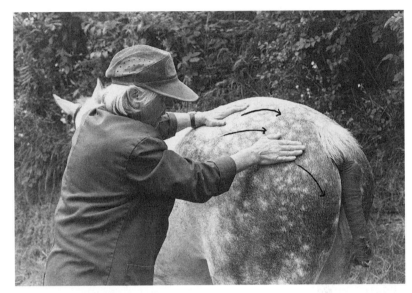

The gluteal mass should be worked from loins to tail, first using effleurage.

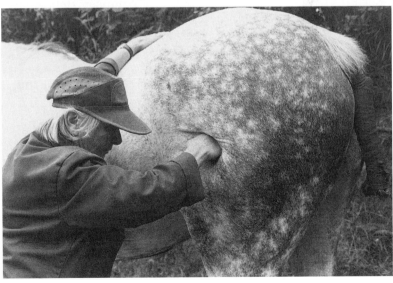

Deep compression over the muscle mass involved in carrying the leg forward.

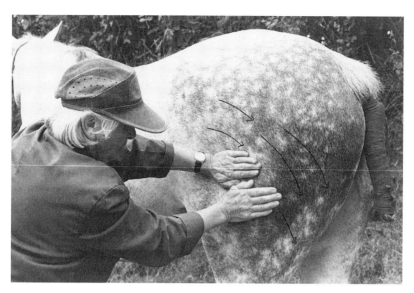

The group of muscles involved in flexing the stifle are worked down and slightly backward.

The muscles of the hindquarter (glutei), influencing the hip joint form a huge rounded mass between the loins, where their fibres intertwine with those of the back musculature, and the tail root. In the average 15.2h animal, these muscles can form a mass some 14in (35.5cm) in depth, creating a need for considerable pressure if massage is to influence the tissues. The group should be worked from the loins towards the tail, first with effleurage, followed by deep compression using a lightly clenched fist or one hand reinforced by the other.

The muscles of the hind limb are more complex in their interaction than those of the forelimb. The groups on the outer side, at the back and the inside of the flank work with the gluteal mass and are all involved in stifle/hock activity. Due to the action of a cable-like muscle, peroneus tertius, these two joints always work as a pair, neither can function independently.

The group of the muscles involved in bringing the limb forward under the body and lying in front of the true hip are worked down and slightly backward from the tubercoccae (point of the hip) towards the inner side of the limb, using effleurage and local compression techniques.

Also involved in all hind-limb activity are the sub-lumbar muscles. The group lie inside the pelvis, extending forward to support the sacroiliac joint and continuing on to be attached in a manner which allows them to assist in flexing the back at the lumbo-sacral junction. These muscles cannot be influenced other than by acupressure, the aim to attempt to relieve discomfort in the case of damage to the sacroiliac joint, or lumbo-sacral junction.

The muscles of the hamstring group, in particular biceps femoris, are very important. Thfois group is worked first along the side of the sacrum, then downward and slightly in, towards the groin. Do not attempt to massage right into the groin area, it is highly sensitive and irritates.

The adductor muscles form the two

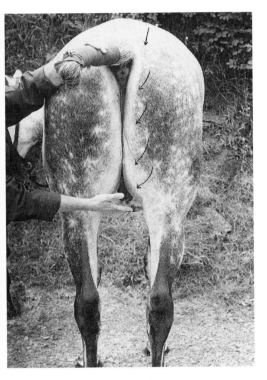

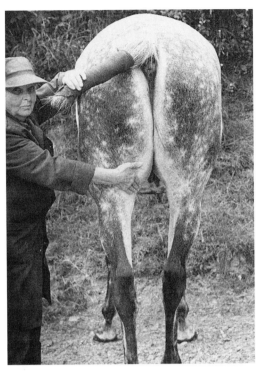

The hamstring group should be massaged along the side of the sacrum, then downward and slightly in towards the groin.

The adductor muscles of the hind limb. The tail is held out of the way in order that the muscle bulk may be clearly seen.

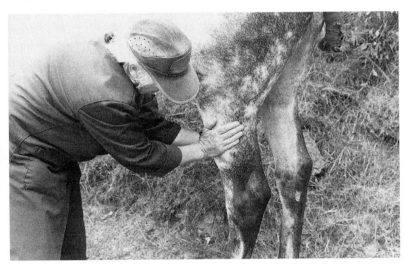

The muscles of the second thigh massed during compression. The second thigh should be worked from the hock upward using inward compression. While the hand position is correct, the hind leg is not resting, making effective massage difficult.

73

cheeks between the hind legs. Normally acting in a stabilizing role, they become active during the lateral work required in dressage. Massage down and forward towards the groin area.

The muscles of the second thigh influence the hock and form the parent muscles of the tendons of the lower leg. Just as in the forelimb, compression using both hands is the best method. Massaging below the hock is unsatisfactory if the leg is lifted and held off the ground. The horse should be taught to rest the hind limb being massaged, as only then will there be sufficient muscle relaxation for the techniques to have any effect.

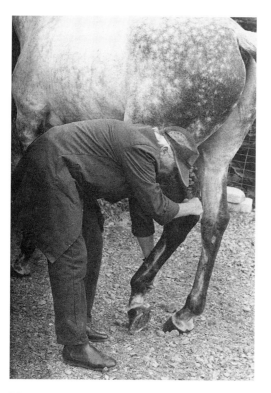

The horse should be taught to rest the limb during massage.

HUMAN SURFACE ANATOMY

Bone Landmarks

Bone points and anatomical landmarks are just as useful in the 'map' of the human body as in the horse, and a thorough understanding of both is essential for successful massage. If no model is available, mapping may be performed on your own body. Other than possibly the mid-back, all areas can be palpated, and using the fingers to identify bone landmarks is an excellent method of touch education.

Head and Neck

Place the index finger of each hand just in front of the ears and open and close the mouth. The movement felt identifies the joint between the lower jaw and the skull, the tempera mandibular joint. Often damaged by the compressive action of the chin strap of a riding helmet, disruption within this joint is the cause of many undiagnosed headaches and migraines.

Using the fingertips of one hand, feel the back of the neck at the point where the head and neck meet. From this area work the fingers downward, centrally. Lying one below the other in a vertical line are a series of bone points; these represent the short spines arising from the seven cervical vertebrae.

At the base of the neck, the last cervical spine C7, projects further than the previous one; this is the area where the neck ends and the chest begins. The enlargement is normal – many people with neck pain imagine they have a swelling in the area, as when they feel for a painful spot they encounter a normal anatomical land-mark and panic.

Shoulders and Chest

The collar bones lie on the front of the chest wall covering the first rib. They are prominent and easily identified. Each joins the shoulder bone of the same side, just above the point of the shoulder.

The scapula lies on the back of the chest wall, the spine superficial, just like that of the horse. The spine can be felt by crossing an arm over the front of the chest, putting the hand over and behind the shoulder and feeling the back of the chest.

These bones, the two scapulae and their conjoined collar bones, create a 'milk-maid's yoke' type structure, sitting over the top of the chest, from which, one at each end, hang the arms.

The sternum, which joins to the clavicle and the first seven pairs of ribs as they curl forward from the spine, is at the centre front of the chest and is felt as a flat bone mass.

The Arm

The head of the humerus lies under the deltoid, a large, inverted, triangular muscle. The upper arm bone is suspended by muscles from the previously described 'yoke'. The head of the humerus is a useful landmark, as the axilla lies between the chest wall and the bone head.

Moving down the arm, the point of the elbow lies at the back of the elbow joint when the palm of the hand is facing forward. With the elbow bent, the tendon of the biceps muscle can be felt lying

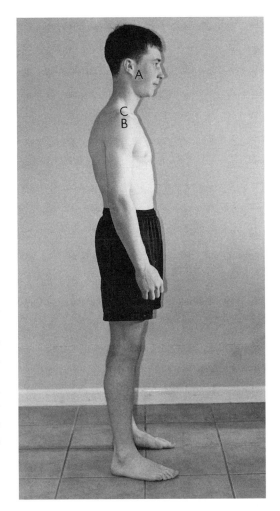

Side view.

A   Tempera mandibular joint, often damaged by the compressive action of the chin strap.

B   Point of shoulder lying just below the junction of collar bone to scapula C, the point of the milk-maid's yoke.

over the front of the joint. Below the elbow two adjacent bones lying in parallel, the radius and ulna, form the forearm, and with their interosseous membrane give

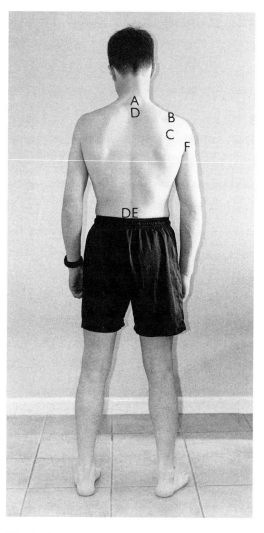

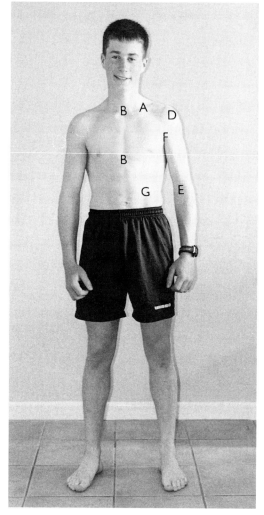

The back.
A   Normal enlargement at C7
B   Spine of the scapular
C   Scapular
DD Line of the posterior spines of the
    12 thoracic vertebrae
DE Junction of last thoracic vertebrae to
    the first lumbar.
F   Back of the axilla, the area towards
    which upper body massage should
    be directed.

Front view.
A   Clavical or collar bone often broken
    if a rider falls onto an outstretched
    hand.
BB Sternum.
D   Deltoid muscle covering the point of
    the shoulder.
E   Tendon of the biceps muscle.
F   The front of the axilla, the area
    toward which upper body massage
    should be directed
G   Last or 12th rib.

origin to the parent muscles of the tendons of the hand.

The two bones of the forearm end at the wrist and may be located with the palm of the hand facing forward. The bone on the thumb side is the distal end of the radius, the bone on the other side is the distal end of the ulna. The tendon of the common digital flexor muscle is palpable between these two points on the palm aspect of the wrist.

The muscles of the arms and shoulders enable the rider to maintain the light contact required between fingers, reins, bit and the horse's mouth. In general this involves isotonic muscle work, with short spells of active contraction. The amount and type of muscle activity will vary, and depends to some extent on the behaviour of the horse – an animal that pulls is more tiring to ride and demands greater muscle activity than a calm, well-schooled animal. The most tiring activity is probably driving a four in hand. Shoulder and arm massage help relax the 'whip' at a three-day event driving competition, enabling control on the third day, cone driving, to be performed with greater sensitivity.

Mid and Low Back

With one hand behind the back, the spines of the twelve thoracic and five lumbar vertebrae can be located lying centrally, one above the other, between the ridges formed by the long mass of the erector spinae muscles.

The human back adopts an 'S' shape when viewed from the side and the subject is vertical, therefore a hollow or concavity in the low back, a convexity in the chest area and a slight concavity in the neck area is normal. The extent of these natural curves varies in each individual.

Pelvis and Leg

The last rib can be felt just above the waist. The upper margin of the front of the pelvic rim can be felt as a distinct bone prominence just below the waist. The distance between the last rib and the pelvic rim varies in each individual, there are no bone landmarks and the area feels soft. The pelvis consists of a ring of bone created from the pelvic bones and the fused sacrum, with the upper body firmly attached at the junction between the last lumbar vertebrae L5 and the first of the fused sacrum S1. The coccyx lies deep between the cheeks of the buttocks.

The top of the femur can be felt on the outer side of the pelvis just above the area where the leg joins the body. Deep to the bone prominence, just as in the horse, lies the hip joint. The patella lies on the front of the knee joint. With the leg supported, in a non-weight-bearing situation, the bone can be pushed from side to side. The knee is designed as a hinge, rotation of the femur on the tibia or vice versa, created by an outside force, can seriously damage the internal components. There are two cruciate ligaments and two cartilages or menisci. The tibia and fibula form the lower leg. At the ankle, the ends of the two bones are plainly visible, the distal end of the tibia on the inner side, the distal end of the fibula on the outer. The two bones grip the talus between them, to form the ankle joint.

MOVEMENT OF THE RIDER

Man is able to ride the horse due to the design of the equine back. The multi-jointed rod, the vertebral column, is supported by muscles and ligaments arranged in a manner that oppose both the downward weight of the abdominal contents and gravitational force. The angle of the ribs as they project laterally from the vertebral column provides a base for the muscle-covered platform upon which the rider sits.

The vertebral column of man is constructed from individual vertebrae: seven cervical; twelve thoracic; and five lumbar, the last of which, L5, is attached to the five fused sacral vertebrae. In man, the coccyx is a vestigial appendage serving no useful purpose. Unfortunately, the small bones are often badly bruised following a fall when the individual lands flat on their seat. (Friction massage is of benefit but is very painful for the subject.) In common with the horse, the human vertebral column is endowed with inter-vertebral discs. However, unlike the horse, these discs are regularly traumatized, leading to pain. The pain is referred to the dermatome of the nerve compressed by the damaged disk. Massage given to the area where the pain is experienced will have little effect, the nerve root needs to be influenced. The choice lies between connective tissue massage (CTM), trigger point massage or acupressure.

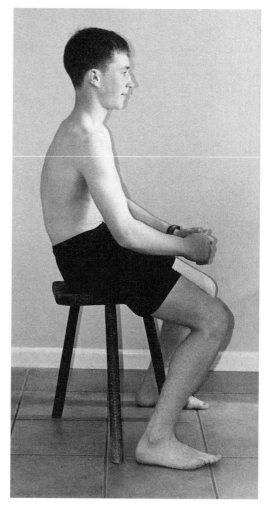

Far too many riders try to rearrange their pelvic angle by realigning their lumbar spine.

The Neck

Composed of seven cervical vertebrae, the neck enjoys multi-axial movement. Range achieved by the interaction of all the vertebrae, other than at the base where the junction of C7 to T1 – an area of maximal movement in the horse – is fixed in man.

The thoracic cage is formed from twelve pairs of ribs, which allows limited bending but considerable twisting or rotation. The ribs perform a bucket-handle movement lifting up to enlarge the chest cavity, then falling back into place. If a horse falls and rolls on to the rider the ribcage

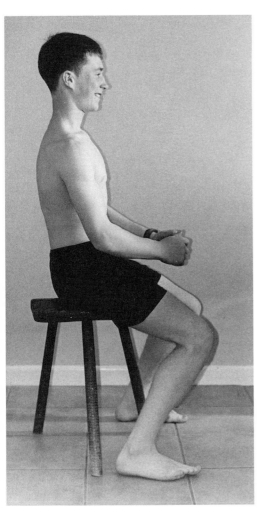

Riders should rearrange the pelvic angle at the hips.

may be compressed and ribs may break. Just as with neck injuries, the situation should be considered a medical emergency. Fractured ribs cause considerable pain: acupressure may help to relieve pain but medical permission must first be obtained.

Mid-back pain is often experienced by riders, often without any identifiable cause. The pain may be secondary to sitting crooked, when the body automatically rearranges its skeletal components to achieve balance. It is also frequently caused when a horse pulls hard or 'rakes'. If this occurs, the muscles running between the thoracic vertebrae and medial border of the scapula are badly over stretched as both arms are wrenched forward. Massage is very helpful, the Swedish techniques being first choice, but it is possible to influence the area using a towel. The towel should be arranged diagonally across the back, one end held above the shoulder, the other end at waist level. Pulling the towel back and forth gives an excellent local massage. Changing the diagonal lie of the towel ensures the whole mid and upper back is targeted.

Low Back, Lumbar Area

Most back problems occur in the lumbar area of the back. The mechanics of this area are not designed to achieve mobility but stability – movement of the upper body on the legs should take place at the hip joints. Unfortunately, the lumbar area is easily stressed. Far too many riders try to rearrange their pelvic angle from above by realigning their lumbar spine, instead of rearranging their pelvic angle at the hips.

Contrary to most beliefs, the jockey rides with the lumbar spine well positioned for security. It is the dressage rider, attempting to angle the pelvis and lumbar spine in order to achieve a 'deep seat', who suffers the most. These riders need help to reduce discomfort and exercise to achieve lumbar stability. Far too many can be seen wobbling like a jelly on their saddles, and in so doing, not only upsetting the balance

79

of their mount, but also increasing the chances of the horse developing a bruised and painful back.

The lumbar spine is designed to angle slightly forward creating a slight concavity, which provides strength and stability. Pain experienced in this area or incorrect balance alignment affects the entire vertebral apparatus. Local massage can be applied using a circular movement with a clenched fist or by pulling a towel back and forth. However, the discomfort will return unless the stresses that created the problem are addressed.

Pain in the back can also arise if the rider has one leg slightly longer than the other. If both stirrup leathers are the same length, the rider will sit crooked, slipping towards the shorter leg. The upper body will compensate by twisting as the balance mechanisms are activated in an attempt to retain an upright posture. The masseur should always check leg length in riders who sit crooked and complain of back pain.

Pelvis

The pelvis consists of a ring of bone created by the arrangement of two pelvic bones and the fused sacrum, the upper body firmly being attached at the junction between L5 and S1. The angle of the 'bone ring' allows the rider to sit on the muscle mass of their buttocks, the mass corresponding to that of the horse's hind quarters.

Hips

The hip joints are of a multi-axial construction, the round ball-like head of the femur attached by an internal ligament to the saucer-shaped socket on the pelvis. The depth of the pelvic socket determines the range of movement at the hip joint – the deeper the socket, the less easy it is to touch the toes during a forward bend, the shallower, the easier. Investigation has shown that many people have lost up to 25

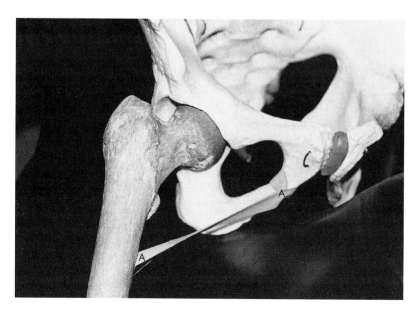

AA, the adductor or 'riders muscles', lie between the inner aspect of the thigh bone and the lowest bone of the pelvic ring, the pubis.

per cent of available hip joint movement simply through lack of activity, stretching in particular. When this occurs the lumbar spine suffers.

The adductor muscle group lies between the inner aspect of the thigh bone and the lowest bone of the pelvic ring, the pubis. This group is often termed 'the rider's muscle', as it acts to retain the position of the thigh bone against the saddle and tears are a common rider injury. Friction and stretching are needed to aid recovery.

For a rider, the hip is the most important of all the body joints, masseurs should ensure their riders are encouraged to mobilize their hip joints following a massage.

Thigh and Knee

The construction of the knee joint, a hinge, is an exact replica of the stifle in the horse, but in man the knee and ankle (stifle/hock) move independently of each other.

The quadricep muscles, running down the front of the thigh, are very active in all riders, initiating and controlling knee movement at trot. The muscles perform concentric work as the knee straightens and the rider's seat leaves the saddle, followed by eccentric work as the rider sits, or work in a static hold if the rider stands in the stirrups.

It is essential to massage these muscles. Sitting relaxed, feet on the floor, knees in mid position, the muscles can be self-influenced by picking up the muscle mass using the palm, thumb and fingers. The area just above the knee joint provides the starting point and the muscle group is worked towards the groin, lifting and releasing the

muscle mass section by section. In the rider, the angle of the knee reflected through the hip joint, determines the position, in particular that of the lumbar area, adopted, to enable the upper body of the individual to remain in balance.

The degree to which the knees need to bend depends upon the discipline. The national hunt and flat jockey will ride with a near fully flexed knee position, the show jumper with slightly less flexion, while the dressage rider is positioned with the knee just off extension.

Ankle

Control, strength and flexibility of the ankle are essential for all riders to enable

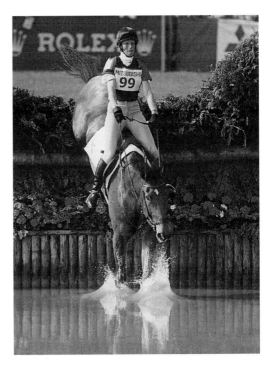

The adductor muscles hold the thighs against the saddle.

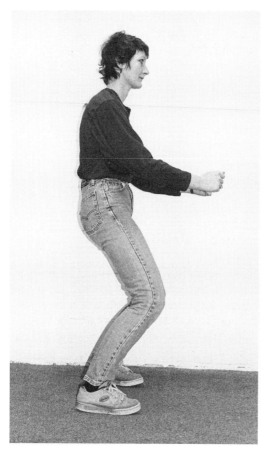

The quadricep muscles running down the front of the thigh are very active in all riding positions.

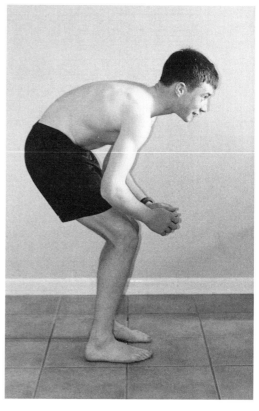

The model simulates the saddle position when jumping or race riding. The position of the hip has altered to one of increased flexion. The quadriceps, in combination with the adductor muscles amd the perenei enable the rider to adopt the position.

them to give correct, positive 'aids'. Stability of the ankle joint is to a large extent provided by the peronei muscles, the group lying on the outer aspect of the calf. In the novice rider these muscles ache, being under-developed for such a demanding role. Massage, particularly CTM, relieves discomfort.

The leather riding boot of the past, afforded extra stability around the ankle, enabling 'the aids' to be applied with minimum effort.

The angle of foot and toe is determined by the position of both the stirrup iron and the knee. If the stirrup does not hang straight, either pushed forward or back by the foot due to an incorrect angle at the knee, the position at the hip will alter, resulting in poor rider balance as the centre of gravity becomes unstable. The resulting inappropriate muscle activity leads to fatigue in the rider and poor performance from the horse.

6 Choice of Method, and Presumed Effects

Before selecting an appropriate method to influence body behaviour it is worth considering a statement made by the late James Cyriax, father of orthopaedic medicine: 'to treat is comparatively easy, it is diagnosis that is difficult'. In order to select the most appropriate and effective massage approach it is important to plan appropriately for the required result.

Virtually no research exists to substantiate any of the claims associated with 'touch'. It is only by considering reactions known to occur following compression of tissue, neural receptors and superficial circulatory vessels that the 'presumed' effects of a touch technique can be suggested. The inter-linkage and inter-dependence of all systems is a fact, so the hypothesis 'what affects one will affect all' is not without foundation.

STIMULATION THROUGH THE USE OF POINTS

Acupressure

As previously discussed in the context of acupuncture or acupressure, the presence of 'points' has recently been scientifically correlated. Some are located at the sites of known neural receptors, while others have been identified due to a specific tissue arrangement following investigation using powerful electron microscopes.

The effects of acupressure are presumed to be the result of neural receptor stimulation. It is beyond the scope of this text to give the exact protocols necessary for the selection of the pertinent points for every acupressure procedure, for in some situations up to fifteen or more points require stimulation to influence an identified problem and ensure a beneficial result. As an example of the complexity of the method, the most recent veterinary text contains over 600 pages of illustration and instruction, of which over 350 pages are devoted to the horse alone. However, despite this in-depth information regarding equine conditions, both medical and surgical, the text contains virtually no specific information concerning disorders of bone and soft tissue. Acupressure and acupuncture must therefore be considered as methods of delivering medical treatment, wider in scope of influence than the conventional Western medical massage approach, but for therapy using these methods in order to be effective and safe, a diagnosis is essential.

STRESS AND TRIGGER POINT MASSAGE

Stress points or trigger points can be likened to *ashi* points. Both Tellington Ttouch and modern shiatsu employ adapted point therapy to influence selected body areas. The masseur working with horse and rider is neither concerned with nor qualified to treat illness in the true sense. Their role is to deal with performance, so their involvement with the body should be confined to musculo-skeletal disorders. To establish an appropriate regime is difficult, for even reference to a renowned human-oriented text, *Essentials of Chinese Acupuncture*, containing information compiled by the Traditional Colleges at Beijing, Shanghai, and Nanjing and used as the main reference source by students at the Acupuncture Institute of the Academy of Traditional Chinese Medicine, is of little help. In this 430-page book, only twenty-two lines of text refer to soft tissue, and even then the main prescription is stated as 'the use of Ashi points'.

Ashi points are considered to be tender or sensitive spots present in certain conditions. They have neither definite described locations, nor, as with acu points, are they named. They are described as follows: 'Where there is a painful spot there is an Ashi point.' In today's terminology these points relate closely to those described as trigger or stress points. The effects of *ashi*, trigger, and stress point stimulation are secondary to the reaction to pressure from local neural receptors. Stimulation of the receptors should activate a natural sequence of events leading to healing and recovery.

Jack Meagher was the first modern-day therapist to describe the use of stress point therapy in the horse, and to successfully adapt and use methods described for the human to treat equine muscle problems. Meagher and other therapists have described points associated with muscle problems and produced charts on which they indicate the location of stress points identified through personal experience. Although charts may act as a useful indicator, the masseur must appreciate that each horse and rider will present differently.

Motor Point Stimulation

The term motor point refers to the command centre of a muscle, a neural complex. These sites are located centrally, within the upper portion of the distal one-third of the muscle belly. Within the structure, motor and sensory fibres command, correlate, communicate and execute; responding, recording and reacting to all manner of stimuli, including those associated with pressure. All the complex chemical interactions involved in muscle activity and behaviour originate within the motor point.

Trigger Points

Myofascial triggers were described in 1992 by Travell and Simons. Their findings defined narrow bands of fibrous tissue laid down within an irritable muscle. They suggested this fibrous reaction appeared to follow an adverse/traumatic situation, which had left an area of muscle ischaemic (lacking in blood).

84

The angle of the fingertip should be vertical, and the pressure directed inward when stimulating motor, stress, trigger, ashi *or* acu *points.*

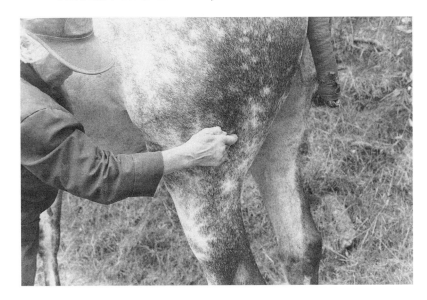

Stress Points

When muscle tissue is replaced by fibrous tissue the tissue is painfully reactive to local pressure. In the Chinese concept this reactive site is obviously that described as an *ashi* point or, in modern terminology, a stress point.

EFFECTS OF STIMULATION

Stimulation of a motor, stress, trigger or *ashi* point activates the normal behavioural characteristics of tissue in response to applied pressure. These reactions, in appropriate circumstances, are beneficial because, for reasons as yet unidentified, damaged tissue seems, in some instances, to be unable to trigger its natural, in-built, healing responses.

To stimulate it is necessary to:

- locate the *ashi*, trigger or stress point;
- place the finger tip, reinforced by a second finger, over the point at an angle that allows a vertical pressure application;
- press inward, maintaining pressure for at least 20–30 seconds;
- at the end of 20–30 seconds release the pressure for 30–40 seconds, then reapply.

As the tissue begins to react to neural messages, activated as a direct response to the pressure, local spasm and sensitivity will reduce. When this occurs stimulation should cease, with a further session, given if required, after a two- or three-day interval.

THE REASON FOR THE CHOICE OF STRESS, OR TRIGGER POINT STIMULATION

If tissue does not repair normally, and should fibrous tissue replace muscle tissue, local contractile efficiency is lost. Unless this contractile property is restored, the affected muscle will, over a period of time, become unable to respond fully to stretch demands, due to repeated micro trauma around the fibrous area.

Loss of muscle mobility results in movement reorganization, and in many instances results in secondary damage elsewhere. For example immobility in the equine trapezius muscle can restrict the forward movement of the forelimb complex. To achieve stride length, shoulder and knee interaction will be modified. In some instances, this being to a degree dependent upon conformation and rider command, stress may be transferred to the muscles at the back of the forelimb. These are the parent muscles of the all-important flexor tendons: tendons forced to extend their length by 10 per cent at speed, and that rely for safety on there being normal properties within their parent muscle. Should this be varied or compromised, extra strain is transmitted to the tendon, often with disastrous results.

Consideration of such a chain of reactions once again establishes the need for the responsible use of massage in a preventive role. Massage, after competition or activity, will, by preventing the formation of adhesions, help to prevent any incorrect fibre replacement and so avoid consequent problems.

Sensitive fingers are necessary to detect the underlying spasm caused by local trauma creating trigger/stress/*ashi* points, as it is only through the sensation of touch, unless a themography unit is available, that these micro lesions can be readily identified.

Motor Points

Anatomical knowledge and accuracy are required to detect motor points. It is also important to understand that direct pressure over the motor point may result in pain in a previously painless area.

Stimulation of the appropriate motor point is used in cases of muscle spasm to achieve relaxation. Spasm reduces circulatory flow and therefore impairs the ability of a muscle to cleanse adequately, to restore supplies of necessary fuel, or to effect recovery following trauma. The technique is exactly as that used for trigger/stress point stimulation.

Meridians

In recent, Western-compiled texts, the spleen – both in man and horse – is considered to rule the muscles, the four limbs and, very logically, the blood. Therefore, when considering methods to influence soft tissue, the spleen meridian deserves consideration. The spleen meridian, in the horse, is considered to start from a point on the inner side of the coronary band, two-thirds of the way forward of the heel bulb. The line continues up the medial aspect of the pastern, angling slightly forward on the cannon, to continue toward the front of the hock, on the medial aspect. From hock to stifle the meridian is medially sited on the tibia, and at the stifle the line angles back toward the tuber coxae. A sharp angulation down and forward along the abdominal wall to the fourth intercostal space continues the line, until at the fourth intercostal space a second sharp angulation occurs, the line angling up and back, ending in the tenth intercostal space at roughly the level of the shoulder joint.

In the human model, the meridian originates on the medial side of the big toe, running along the medial aspect of the foot

The spleen meridian in the horse is considered to rule the muscles, the four limbs and the blood.

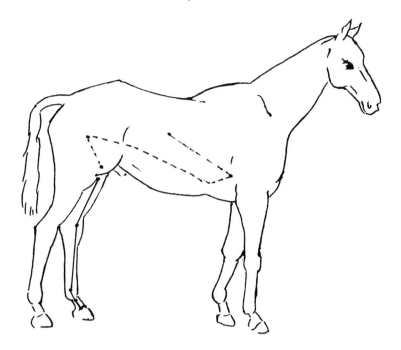

to continue up the lower limb to the medial aspect of the knee, travelling medially from there up the tibia to the groin. In the groin an angulation is present, before the line continues along both the abdominal and chest walls. In the upper portion of the chest it is considered to become deep, following the line of the throat to end beneath the tongue.

Stimulation of points along the meridian *should* influence muscles, circulation and limb-associated problems.

Opening Meridians

A major descriptive link between Chinese methods and techniques currently in use becomes apparent when describing Swedish effleurage. The method used for 'the opening of meridians to influence the flow of Chi energy' is described as 'allowing the hands to glide smoothly over the body surface in line with the meridians'. This is an exact replication of effleurage, used to prepare tissues prior to the application of any of the additional techniques included in a Swedish routine.

There are many factors to consider. The location of a stress point within a muscle will vary. Local discomfort is caused by tissue changes, secondary to activity-induced stress. Each activity will stress different muscle groups and different areas within an individual muscle. Gait, speed, a fall or a slip may influence the area of fibre damage. The conditioning of the musculature, the state of the ground and the cardio-vascular efficiency must be considered prior to selection of site and technique, for all have a direct influence. While the site for therapy application will alter, the changes within the tissues following mechanical stress will not vary.

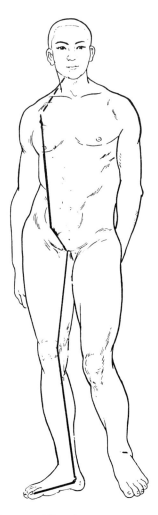

The spleen meridian in man is considered to rule the muscles, the four limbs and the blood.

Disruption of normal tissue architecture results in:

- cellular breakdown;
- inter-cellular fluid leakage from the damaged tissue cells into the extra-cellular fluid;
- the resultant adverse chemical situation being reported to the brain by local nerve centres and appropriate reparative steps instigated;
- the damaged local circulatory vessels are sealed off; those undamaged constrict to prevent possible fluid loss;
- reduction of local circulation;
- tissue fluids, including lymph, migrate to the area to scavenge debris;
- pain occurs, both insult pain and pain secondary to increased local pressure;
- the area, if palpated, causes a pain reaction from the subject; and
- tension in adjacent muscle tissue causes local spasm, futher reducing circulation.

Areas of damage can, with experience, be detected by the discerning masseur and the appropriate technique applied to retain mobility of the damaged area. Tissue reconstruction should occur naturally; but if the area is traumatized repeatedly, a chronic situation occurs, with fibrous rather than normal tissue laid down. In such cases a more aggressive approach, such as friction massage, may be required and a reason for the repeated traumatization sought.

Considerations Regarding Choice of Method

Trigger points detected, following known trauma or perceived activity-induced stress, respond well to massage. However, stress or myofascial trigger points must be carefully considered lest they are the result of referred pain. That is pain arising elsewhere in the body mass but reflected, through a common nerve pathway, to the appropriate dermatome. In such situa-

ions care must be exercised as concen-
trated stimulation, applied to very
localized areas or points, can, in the
absence of a diagnosis or if the effects are
not properly understood, be detrimental
rather than useful.

CONNECTIVE TISSUE MASSAGE (CTM)

Connective tissue massage is a specialist
technique extending beyond the confines
of point usage by influencing entire
areas or zones, considered to be associated
with underlying bands of connective
tissue.

Connective tissue, also called fascia,
is present throughout the body mass
and, as the name suggests, functions as
a contiguous interconnection between
all individual segments that form the
whole. Immensely strong, although when
viewed at dissection appearing thin
and translucent, the tissue suspends,
along with a plexus of blood and lymphatic
vessels, many types of nerve endings
(neural receptors). This fact is pertinent
to the masseur, for by working along
prescribed tissue interfaces extensive
neural stimulation is achieved.

CTM is considered to:

- rebalance sympathetic and parasympathetic nerve interaction;
- reduce fascial tension;
- improve visceral function;
- influence and balance hormonal and
  endocrine function;
- promote fluid level balance;
- improve circulatory flow;
- reduce referred pain sensation;
  and
- promote a feeling of relaxation.

The methods of application, described in
the Connective Tissue chapters of professional massage books, mirror the
techniques now variously described under
the titles Skin Rolling, Bowen Technique,
Shiatsu and Ttouch, so it is reasonable to
suggest that the effects can only be
similar.

SKIN ROLLING AND BOWEN TECHNIQUE

Skin Rolling and Bowen require that,
using one or both hands, a fold of skin is
lifted gently upward and held as a 'roll'
between fingers and thumb. The fingers
continuously move the fold in a way
which ensures that as the far side of the
roll is released and returns to its normal
position, the near-side skin is lifted, so
retaining the desired roll. The skin is
therefore manipulated in a way that
achieves a wave-like traction effect on
the connective tissue/fascial layer
beneath. The effect is stimulation of
neural receptors.

Shiatsu, Ttouch

The stimulus is one of light touch, pressure applied using either the tips of
the fingers or thumbs, these moved to
small circles along the length of the chosen
connective tissue zone, or by pressing
gently down over the extent of the zone
using fingers or thumbs. The effects of
Connective Tissue Massage (CTM), the
Bowen Technique and Tteam are neural:
the techniques influence the neural
plexus of the connective tissue matrix,
and follow meridians if applied throughout zones.

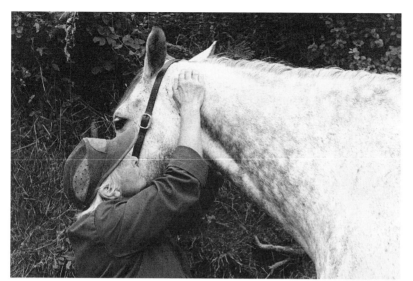

The fingers of one hand are closed lightly together and describe a series of small circular movements along a zone.

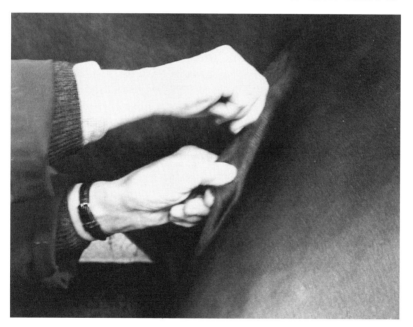

Techniques for skin rolling or Bowen. A fold of skin is lifted upward between fingers and thumbs.

Acupressure, trigger, stress point and motor point therapy employ localized deep pressure applied at a predetermined site or sites, these selected following consideration of problems deduced and the results required.

Tteam and Shiatsu are sometimes confined to stimulation in a local sense, but may use the zone approach.

MASSAGE DEVICES

Before considering Swedish massage in depth, massage devices require consideration. A number of massage devices are commercially available. Designed either as a pad or with small, rounded applicators, they are either run from mains electricity or are battery powered. The devices are designed, when held or strapped in place, to produce vibrations and to transfer these deep into the underlying tissue masses. The frequency of the vibrations has been carefully calculated to influence the natural pain responses of the body in line with information supplied by Melzac and Wall. In their *Gate Theory of Pain* they describe the effects on neurones of cyclical vibrations of set frequency, delivered in a manner that ensures a constant cyclical repetition over a prescribed time. Their research demonstrates a reduction in the ability of pain receptors to record if subjected to correctly calculated vibration stimuli. Reduced pain leads to a reduction of local muscle spasm, allowing a restoration of circulatory flow and so enhancing recovery.

In the case of the horse it may be debatable if it is sensible to totally remove pain. All pain is present for a reason and the horse is unable to describe discomfort. Removal of pain allows the animal to move without restriction, for the natural guarding mechanism afforded by the pain response is no longer operational. This situation may not be beneficial. Hand massage will subdue, but not totally remove, pain, particularly if the origin of the pain is sited in deep structures.

Magnetic Massagers

Hand-held magnetic devices, containing two small, magnetized steel balls set side by side and which revolve as the device is pushed back and forth over muscle masses, are claimed to restore the normal energy balance in damaged tissue. Norfields USA, who have commissioned more research into the effects of magnetism on tissue than most manufacturers, have recently designed a hand-held, battery operated, vibrating magnetic device, thus incorporating pain relief through cyclical repetition and energy rebalance from the magnetic field.

Tennis Ball Massage

Large muscle masses, hard to influence by hand, can be massaged by using a tennis ball. The ball is placed over the target area and, using considerable pressure, is rolled or twisted in a circular manner. The effects are of intermittent compression.

Massage Gloves

A variety of skin stimulating/massage gloves are available. These do little more than achieve minimal skin stimulation with a consequent local hyperaemia.

While no device should be condemned, none can replicate hand massage, the most obvious reason being the total lack of feedback achieved through the operator's hands. The techniques in the method of touch known as Swedish massage provide the basics for several of the routines offered by the masseur.

SWEDISH MASSAGE

The procedures employed in Swedish massage obviously overlap with other methods using touch, but the effects achieved are unlikely to create adverse reactions within the subject, as the techniques are designed for general, rather than specific influence and should always be considered as a first choice.

Swedish massage describes and embraces all classic massage techniques; every other form of massage described includes one or more of the Swedish methods of hand or finger application. The techniques are also the basis of sport massage, lymphatic drainage, sport lymphatic drainage and aromatherapy.

The aims of Swedish massage are to:

- maintain a stable state within a body;
- achieve a state of relaxation, both local and general;
- influence and enhance venous and lymphatic flow;
- improve tissue fluid interchange;
- prepare the body for activity;
- assist in the removal of chemical irritants present in muscle following activity;
- enhance general body recovery, post-activity;
- in cases of tissue damage, enhance normal recovery; and
- ensure healing is by first intent, by retaining tissue mobility and minimizing the risk of scarring and/or adhesions.

Dependent upon body area, muscle bulk, shape and size of the subject, the masseur has several choices at their disposal. They may choose to use: one hand, the second used in a supporting role to give a feeling of security; both hands working in parallel or alternately; the fingers; a single finger, which may be reinforced by a second; or the thumb or thumbs.

In order to ensure maximum benefit, the tissues should be worked, as far as possible, in parallel with venous blood flow, returning as it does toward collection centres in both the groin and axilla. In the horse, hair lie must be considered and may necessitate modification of the ideal direction.

It is essential to retain rhythm in order to promote relaxation, and also to transfer smoothly, without loss of contact, from one technique to another.

EFFLEURAGE

Effleurage is described as a 'stroke' and is the first, interlinking and final technique in all Swedish-based massage routines. The technique can be double-, alternate- or single-handed; the hands are moulded to the underlying contour and should execute a series of long, slow, rhythmical strokes.

In the double-handed technique both hands work simultaneously. In the alternate-handed technique, as one hand completes a stroke the second, appropriately re-positioned, begins a stroke. In the single-handed technique one hand works while the second supports.

The strokes should commence away from, or distal to, the body centre, the

Effleurage – a long sweeping rhythmic application.

(Top) Single-handed effleurage - the second hand used in a supporting role.

(Bottom) Double-handed effleurage of the neck.

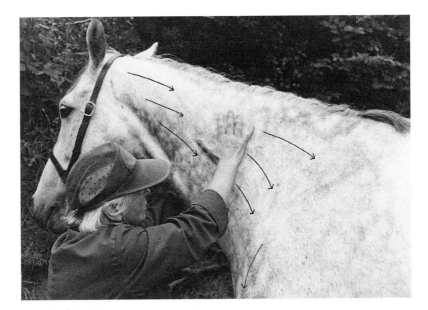

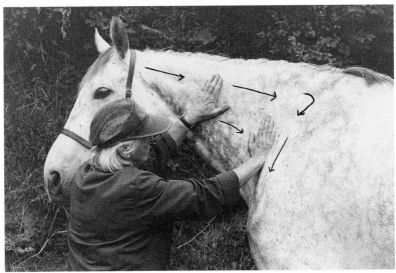

hands working segmentally toward either the axilla or groin. At the end of a stroke the hands should be moved lightly over the surface and repositioned for the next stroke. As an area is worked, subsequent strokes should be performed in a manner and direction that ensures overlap of the previously targeted area. Contact should be firm but light until relaxation occurs. Pressure can then be increased, with care taken not to create discomfort by working powerfully over superficial structures such as the spine of the scapular. The effects of slow

93

rhythmical strokes with sustained pressure achieve general relaxation, rapid strokes stimulate.

There is a natural opiate release within 'rubbed' tissues leading to a reduction of local pain or discomfort (the natural reaction is to 'rub' an area that hurts).

PETRISSAGE

Petrissage is described as a compressive technique using finger compression. Kneading and wringing influence deep-sited tissue. When kneading pressure is applied vertically inward over the target area, and as the tissues deform and the required depth is achieved the operating hand or body part is moved in a manner that achieves an upward sweep accompa-

nied by pressure release. The technique is continued by exact replication of the movement over the adjacent area.

The method of application may be executed using: one hand; both hands; one hand reinforced by the second; an elbow; or a clenched fist. The choice is determined by the tissue mass of the target area. When the technique is appropriate in small, localized areas the pads of the fingers are used.

Wringing is a double-handed compression technique almost impossible to use on a horse but useful when working on a person. The hands work as a pair grasping a roll of muscle tissue. Holding the roll between fingers and thumb, one hand is moved away from the other and toward the masseur, twisting the tissue. The tissue is released and the adjacent segment 'wrung'. The masseur's hands

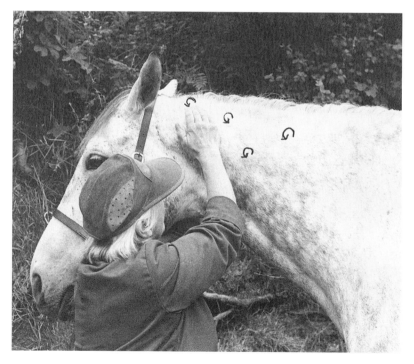

Petrissage. A compression technique. The technique may be double or single handed, or the fingertips may be used. Pressure is applied inward and out using a circular movement. Press in, rotate slightly maintaining pressure, relax and rotate reducing pressure, lift out.

94

work along the fibre direction of the target muscle.

The effects of these techniques are to replicate artificially pressure changes within tissue, which occur naturally during muscle activity. Other than arterial blood, which is subjected to the pressure created by each heart beat, fluids and cells rely on chemical messengers and tissue pressure changes for mobility.

TAPOTMENT

Tapotment is a double-handed technique that stimulates underlying tissue. The

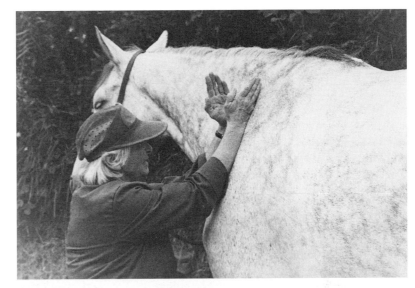

Hacking – a stimulatory technique. Rotation of the forearm allows alternating contact between outer edge of the hand and the underlying tissue.

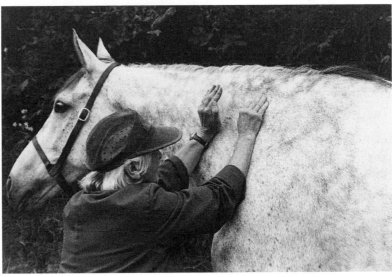

Clapping – a stimulatory technique with the hands held in a 'cup'.

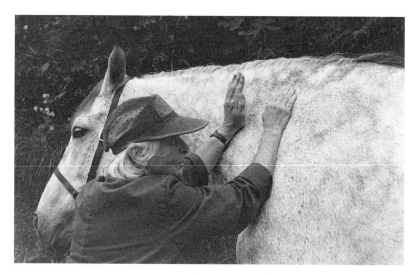

The hands are incorrect: they are not correctly cupped so a slap will result

use of the sides of the hands constitutes 'hacking', the use of the palms 'clapping'. To perform either hacking or clapping the forearms are held at right angles to the body. Both techniques should be performed in a brisk, rapid manner, using very light contact, the hands never stationary but continuously moving over the body surface.

Hacking employs the little-finger sides of the hands. The hands are placed side-by-side over the target area. The action required is obtained by a rotation of the wrist, the movement lifting the side of the hand upward then allowing it to drop. The hands alternate during the technique.

In clapping, each hand is formed into a relaxed 'cup' by drawing the thumb toward the little finger. The fingers are straight but held with slight bending, or flexion, of the knuckles. The hands are placed side by side. The movement required occurs at the wrist, one hand being lifted upward and then dropped to make light contact. As one hand makes the downward movement the other is lifted, ensuring the hands rise and fall in

an alternate manner. The contact should be light yet brisk, the masseur taking care to avoid slapping. If the hand position is correctly formed, air is trapped between the curved palm and the skin, resulting in a hollow sound at contact.

FRICTION

Friction differs from other techniques, as the required effect is to irritate the area targeted in order to break down tissue to re-establish the natural healing reaction of the body.

The technique is applied by using the tip of one finger reinforced by a second; the digit is moved in either a very small circular, or transverse manner. The skin must move as one with the underlying targeted tissue. The placement remains the same for the entire treatment session and the direction employed is aimed at working across the lie of the tissue architecture, rather than in parallel, as is the case in all other techniques.

Friction massage. The movement is performed across the fibre lie.

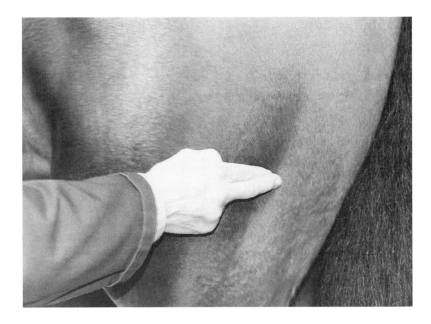

A session of at least fifteen minutes is required for the technique to be effective. Friction massage should be selected for the following:

- to irritate tissue to stimulate local circulation in conditions of chronic recurring injury;
- to break down adhesions;
- to mobilize deep scarring; and
- to mobilize adherent tissue interfaces.

GUIDELINES

An understanding of the probable effects of the differing techniques allows choice, but whichever method is selected the following guidelines are suggested:

- Arrange the subject in surroundings that ensure comfort and safety for subject and masseur.
- The venue should be chosen with the requirement for relaxation of the subject in mind.
- Identify areas of discomfort.
- Select an appropriate regime.
- Consider the time available.
- If a full body massage is needed, allow an hour.

CONTRAINDICATIONS

There are two quotes that those involved in therapy should remember: 'if in doubt, keep out', and 'better to be safe than sorry'. Massage should not be given in any of the following situations:

- Immediately after an accident.
- Following an accident with suspected haemorrhage. Use ice and compression, request professional assistance.
- If there is persistent undiagnosed pain.

- In situations when the subject is dehydrated.
- If there is any type of general or local infection, including undiagnosed fever.
- In a case where any type of skin disruption, fungal or bacterial infection of the skin is present, including rain scald.
- Over an open wound or in areas of active bone growth. (In the early stages of healing local massage is sometimes requested, but proceed with caution.)

- In cases with colic.
- In cases of 'tying up'.
- To remove acute pain/discomfort during competition without veterinary or medical agreement.

As all the techniques are directed primarily at retaining/restoring mobility, therapy sessions should be followed by passive movements, if the area can be thus influenced, or otherwise by actively exercising the muscles involved.

7 Passive Movements, Passive Stretches and Active Exercises

A joint is the meeting place of two or more individual bones. The joints involved in movement are encapsulated, unlike those between the individual bones forming the skull. Described as synovial joints, the specialist tissue enveloping the bone ends and their opposing articular surfaces, functions to restrain movement to that appropriate for the joint shape, and to retain the all-important lubricant, synovial fluid, between the articular surfaces of the joint.

On the outer aspect of the capsule, ligaments span individual joints. Their arrangement affords support to the joint and restricts movement to an appropriate range. These external ligaments work in close partnership with adjacent muscle groups. The muscles create joint movement but can also function to support and stabilize.

Each joint has a range of movement specific to its anatomical construction – a hinge joint is capable of movement in one plane, while a ball-and-socket joint is capable of multi-axial movement.

Joints are loaded with neural sensors that monitor the joint and are in constant communication with the brain and all the other structures and systems involved in joint function, including muscle and ligament.

Passive movements, passive stretches or active exercises should always follow a massage when the tissues are warm. A passive movement is a joint movement performed without any muscular involvement on the part of the subject. The joint or joints are moved by the masseur through their normal anatomical range held in a non weight-bearing position.

A passive stretch moves a joint or joints in exactly the same manner as that used for a passive movement, but at the end of range, over-pressure marginally increases range so stretching all involved structures, capsule, ligaments and muscles.

An active movement is a movement in response to muscle activity, the range of which is restricted by muscle flexibility and conformation. People who have always experienced difficulty in touching their toes, even as children, usually have a deeper hip socket acetabulum than others; just as some horses have a straighter shoulder than others. The rider with a deep hip socket will not have a range of movement comparable to the rider with a shallow socket. Massage can do nothing to influence this – it is a matter of conformation. However, even within these limitations, stretching will help to achieve a greater movement range.

Whilst certain of the joints of the appendicular skeleton can be passively moved through their full range, stretching can only be actively performed in the joints of the axial skeleton.

Why Stretch?

Flexible muscles are essential for economic activity – tight, non-flexible muscles restrict the range of movement, resulting in fatigue and areas of the body being subjected to inappropriate demands.

Whilst it is important to incorporate stretching in workout routines to retain an overall suppleness, care should always be taken to avoid discomfort caused by overstretching. Pain is not the objective, stretching is aimed at restoring or maintaining a normal range of movement and muscle flexibility.

Preparation and Safety

- The tissues should be warm and relaxed before being stretched.
- Tissues should always be prepared for stretching if the movements are to be performed by a masseur. Active stretching is controlled by proprioceptive reflexes which resist inappropriate movement.

- The normal range and plane of movement must be understood and appreciated.
- The limb must be held in a manner that allows the masseur to be comfortable and ensures that contradictory messages from the joints of the limb are avoided. For example, if the fetlock joint is supported rather than allowed to drop and move towards extension, the proprioceptive signals to all other joints associated with extension to prepare for a coordinated movement response will be reduced.
- Move the joints slowly – if resistance is felt, reposition and try again.
- Repeat each movement three to five times. This is adequate.

THE RIDER

Hip flexibility is the key to a safe, effective seat. The group of muscles often described as the 'rider's muscles' are the hip adductors. Running from the femur to the symphysis of the pelvis, the hip adductors pull the leg inward and act as the principal muscles of grip.

New cavalry recruits used to be lunged bareback in order to strengthen their adductor muscles and teach them to balance. To retain balance and flexibility, it is no less important today for riders to stretch their adductor muscles regularly.

Adductor Stretch

The adductor stretch should be an active not a passive stretch in case the muscle, which is in part fibrous, is torn by overpressure.

The adductor stretch. AA indicates the site of the muscles being actively stretched.

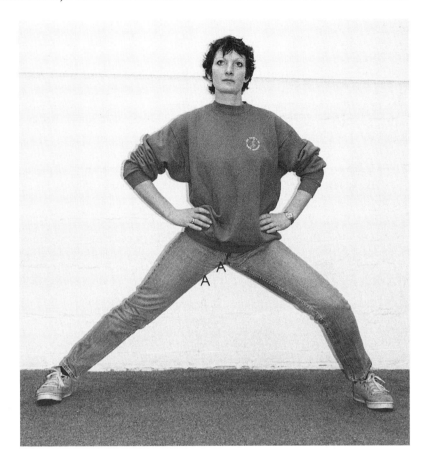

- Take a stride stance holding the upper body vertical.
- Move the upper body sideways until the knee towards which the body moves is forced to bend.
- Continue to move the body weight towards the bent knee until the inner side of the opposite leg begins to register a feeling of stretch just below the groin.
- Hold the position for approximately 10–15 seconds, then swing the body back centrally and outward the opposite way until the feeling of stretch is felt in the leg previously bent at the knee.

- Achieve a rhythm – swing out to one side, hold; swing centrally; swing out to the opposite side, hold.

Never overstretch by continuing for too long. Until the area feels flexible, a set of ten repetitions performed on a daily basis is adequate. Once flexibility has been achieved, a single weekly session will retain the improvement.

Hip Extensor Stretch

The second set of hip muscles to stretch are those lying behind the joint, the hip extensors (glutei). Any limitation of hip flexion,

101

however slight, caused by lack of extensibility in the hip extensors, will affect the low back. These muscles, the buttock muscles, will benefit from passive stretching after activity or a massage when the tissues are warm. The active stretch should be performed on a firm surface such as a massage couch or the floor – a bed is too soft.

- Lie flat on the back with legs straight. Grasp one knee. Pull the leg, bent at

hip and knee, gently towards the chest until the thigh meets the chest wall.

The second leg should, if the hip extensors are flexible, remain flat against the underlying surface. If the straight leg begins to bend, lifting off the underlying surface, hip flexibility in the hip of the leg being pushed toward the chest is poor and will affect rider position. This stretch should be repeated three or four

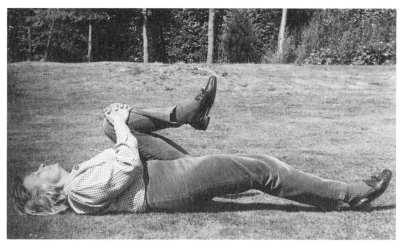

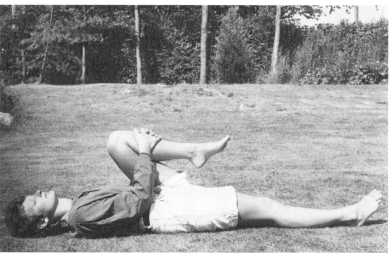

Hip mobility.

Top plate demonstrates tight gluteal muscles, the straight leg is beginning to flex at the knee.

Bottom plate demonstrates a flexible hip, the straight leg remains in contact with the ground.

The muscles are stretched by pulling the leg gently toward the chest in the same position as that used for testing the mobility.

times a session and continued until the second leg remains in contact with the underlying surface as the contralateral limb is flexed on to the chest.

Once restored, the following exercise will ensure that flexibility is maintained.

- Lie flat on the back with one knee towards the chest. Grasp the bent leg below the knee and pull the leg on to the chest.

Riders should not attempt to do this unassisted as they will, without realizing it, change the position of their low back (lumbar spine), creating a damaging flexion in the area.

THE HORSE

Passive movement is useful in arthritic conditions and following sesamoid trauma. At the conclusion of each movement or set of movements, reposition the limb with the horse. Do not let the animal snatch or stamp down.

Passive Neck Stretch

Horses that fall on to their heads tend to 'telescope' their necks, often substantially reducing flexibility. Active neck stretching does not always help. The following passive neck stretch is often effective and one that

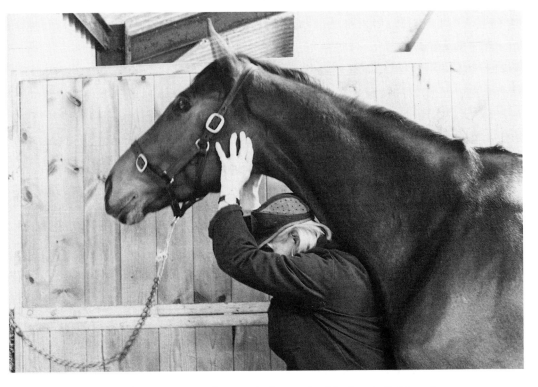

Passive neck stretch. The masseur pushes gently forward achieving a slight neck stretch in a longitudinal plane.

a horse will sometimes allow if sufficiently relaxed following a neck massage.

- Stand under the neck of the horse, buttocks against the front of the animal's chest, with the horse's neck resting over the centre of the back.
- The hands cup the angles of the horse's jaw and the fingers rub the cheek (masseter) muscles until the horse relaxes.
- Push gently forward to produce a slight neck stretch in a longitudinal plane.

Active Neck Stretches

Flexion	Bending the head between the front legs.
Side Flexion	Turning the head sideways in both directions towards the flank. The muzzle should reach the end of the ribcage, even the flank. A horse that rotates the head early in the movement requires continued sessions of neck massage to release tight muscles.

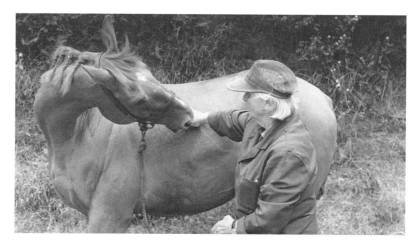

Side flexion demonstrating a mobile neck.

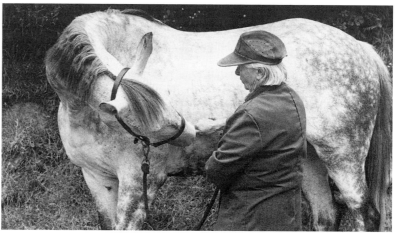

Side flexion demonstrating a stiff neck. The horse has both lowered his head and rotated in an attempt to follow the treat.

Extension Lifting the head. This important movement is all too often overlooked.

Some form of gastronomic inducement is usually needed to persuade the horse to move the neck as required!

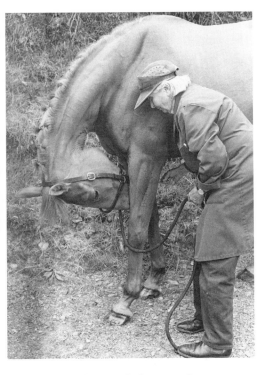

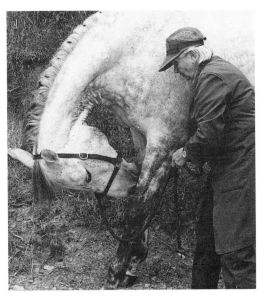

The horse is unable to reach between the front legs and has stretched the near forelimb forward in an attempt to reach the treat.

The horse reaches easily between the front legs.

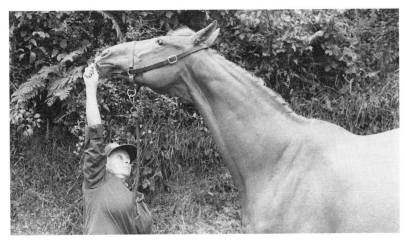

Extension.

Passive Forelimb Movements and Stretches

A stretch should be performed with great care, always taking conformation into account. For example, a horse habitually standing over at the knee will be very uncomfortable if that knee is forced to full extension. The holds and positioning are identical for both movements and stretches. The procedures, be they movements or stretches, should be performed in a manner that mirrors normal movement in both range and plane.

- Pick the limb up as though the foot is to be cleaned.
- Gently push the limb under the body. This stretches the muscles in front of the withers, at the base of the neck, and over the front of the shoulder complex.
- Pull the limb, still in flexion, forward. The knee can be fully flexed, still supported, after stretching the shoulder and elbow.

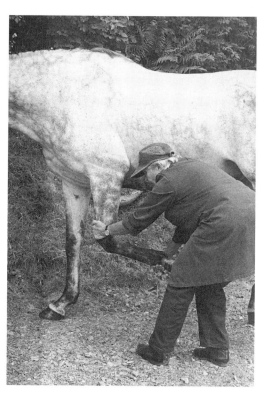

The knee is brought back into flexion and carried back under the body. The fetlock is supported mirroring the natural angulation to avoid contradictory proprioceptive neural massage. Pressure to achieve the movement is applied above the knee, NOT directly over the joint.

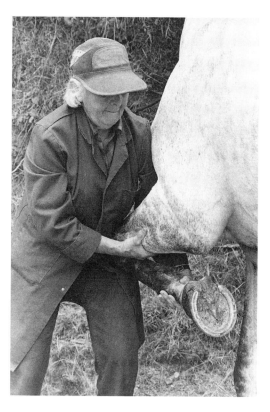

The leg is picked up as though the foot is to be cleaned. The fetlock can be fully flexed with the limb supported thus. The fetlock will not extend as in active action.

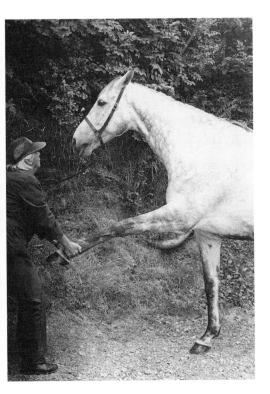

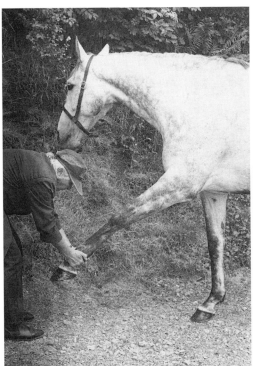

Above: *The horse is showing apprehension, the ears show this. The limb is too high. Incorrect.*

Above: *A comfortable position for the horse. Correct. For a full leg stretch the limb is taken forward of the body in a low position. The fetlock is supported in mid position mirroring the natural angulation of active movement. This avoids contradictory proprioceptive neural messages.*

With the knee in flexion a small amount of passive internal and external motion is possible at the joint. However, unless there are known to be internal adhesions within the joint restricting normal range, the benefits of these movements are debatable.

- The leg is carried forward of the body in a lowered position in order to stretch the entire limb. This is another movement to stretch the muscles in front of the withers, at the base of the neck, and over the front of the shoulder complex.
- The knee is brought back into flexion so that the leg may be carried back under the body and lowered before being positioned straight. This is another movement to stretch the muscles behind the withers, the adductors, and the muscles of the elbow.

At the conclusion of each movement, or set of movements, reposition the limb with the horse, do not let the animal snatch or stamp down.

107

Passive Hind Limb Movements and Stretches

The hind limb is moved as a whole. Other than the fetlock, isolation of movement to a part of the limb is not possible. Given the possibility that the horse may kick, the masseur must take great care in selecting the safe position – the force of a kick increases with distance.

- The limb is picked up as though the foot is to be cleaned, the fetlock held as near to mid-position as the horse will allow.
- The limb is carried forward under the

*Right and below:
Passive stretches,
the hind limb. The
leg is picked up and
with the fetlock in
the normal anatom-
ical position the leg
is taken forward
under the body.*

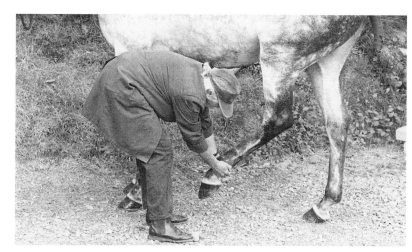

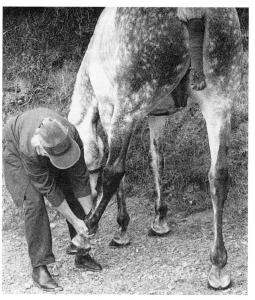

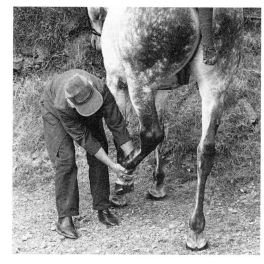

(Above) *Correct.*
(Left): *Incorrect, the leg is being taken outside
the normal movement line.*

108

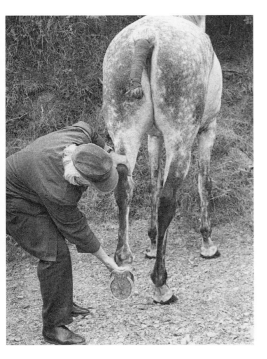

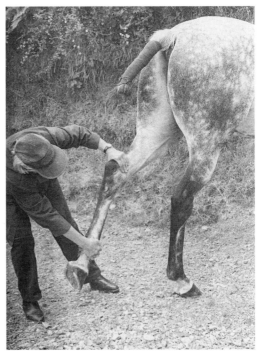

Incorrect hold, the fetlock is stretched and downward pressure on the hock is being used to straighten the limb.

The leg is taken behind the body. Note the fetlock is held positioned as in normal active motion at each stage of the movement. The hock is not pushed straight, but grasped in a manner which ensures the horse is unable to kick violently.

body mass. The muscles stretched are those of the hind quarters and all those lying from the tail root to the hock.

A major mistake is for the masseur to take the leg out to the side. This pulls on the adductor groups and causes the horse, receiving warning signals of incorrect limb positioning, to struggle.

- The limb is carried out behind the horse. The muscles stretched are those lying in front of the hip joint and those controlling the stifle.
- The limb is repositioned with active participation from the horse, the hock point continuing to be grasped until the limb is on the ground.

Grasping the point of the hock firmly prevents the horse kicking violently and is an essential safety precaution.

Lateral Movements

Although required in dressage, lateral movements are not naturally performed by the horse. While some degree of passive abduction and adduction can be performed by the therapist replication of correct active movement is impossible. Active exercises in hand are the best way to

109

retain or restore the movements, the horse being persuaded to move sideways using the limbs correctly. Backing up in hand is also a useful exercise.

Pressure over reflex points will initiate active dorsi, ventro and lateral flexion of the back from withers to loins but the best way to influence the back is to allow the horse space to roll. Postural muscle tone becomes minimal when the horse is on the ground allowing the vertebral column to realign naturally.

Tail Circling

Remarkably little is written about the tail. If observing horses it is quite obvious that the tail is moved during motion, more by some horses than others. Tail circling appears to relax the hind quarters and the loins, particularly if preceded by point massage on either side of the tail root. If the horse is known to kick, tail circling is best performed over a stable door.

The horse, held by an assistant, is backed up to a door. The masseur stretches over the door, first rubbing the hind-quarter muscles then working either side of the tail. Once the horse is relaxed, the tail should be grasped, comfortably yet firmly, and circled first one way and then the other.

Right: *The tail is grasped and held out from the body, as the horse becomes accustomed to both hold and position the masseur circles the tail towards himself. The tail is replaced in its normal position, the masseur changes sides and repeats the circling. DO NOT stand directly behind the horse unless working over a closed stable door.*

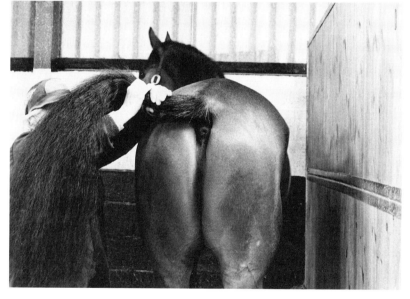

8 Massage for Horse and Rider

MUSCULAR FATIGUE

Studies conducted on both man and the horse demonstrate that factors associated with fatigue are very often present throughout the body musculature for at least one to three days following heavy or unaccustomed activity. In man, sensations of stiffness and pain in the muscles and joints are frequently experienced following bouts of exercise. Changes in gait at walk and trot are obvious in the horse – this usually described as 'pulling out stiff'. A disinclination to exercise or perform as required and a temporary loss of normal performance capability may be observed in both species. While the use of positive thinking may go some way to compensate for performance loss in man, a horse will prove more difficult to motivate, particularly if it is dehydrated.

Research has examined metabolic changes in muscle following activity, and changes in pH along with lactate accumulation have been identified as being responsible for muscle pain. Abnormal muscle membrane conductance, disturbance of the body immune system, and longstanding viral infections have also been shown to have a significant influence on muscle performance and recovery. Recent research has established that travelling increases body stress, leading to fatigue. However, it is known those mentioned above are not the only causative factors – the full extent of the reasons for fatigue have still to be identified.

If the body is in a state of exercise-induced fatigue, secondary to any of the identified situations, the processes to promote recovery will be naturally induced. For the masseur to interfere by stimulating neurones, so introducing contradictory signals can seriously delay recovery.

Dehydration

Electrolytic balance is very important. Interestingly, horses evaluated for fatigue in an endurance study demonstrated a persistent decrease in body weight for several days following a fifty-mile ride. The animals were shown to have re-established normal plasma volume levels (blood fluid) but had developed a generalized body water deficit due to electrolyte replacement failure and so were unable to rebalance their total body fluid content.

Dehydrated animals will not benefit from massage and the possibility of dehydration must always be ruled out before massage is given. Every masseur should know how to establish whether a horse is dehydrated by using the skin pinch test. A fold of skin on the neck is lifted up and held between finger and thumb for 10 to 15 seconds. When released, the skin should immediately return to its normal position, not remain as a raised fold.

Inadequate Oxygen Supply

Both respiratory and cardio-vascular conditions will have a direct influence on muscle behaviour, as a supply of oxygen is critical for sustained activity. Restriction of chest expansion due to the confines imposed by some body protectors reduces oxygen uptake and can lead to increased rider fatigue, a factor ignored by many.

Exercise Induced Pulmonary Haemorrhage (EIPH)

Care must be taken with horses known to bleed following exercise and it must be understood that these animals will take considerably longer to regain pre-activity performance. Many present with marked spasm in the muscles of both back and loins following an episode of EIPH. Massage may reduce the spasm but the relaxation achieved reverses, in the author's experience, within two or three hours.

Degenerative Diseases

Certain conditions, many not fully understood, result in muscle wasting. If this should occur, the remaining muscle tissue becomes overloaded, resulting in early fatigue.

Excess Body Weight

In man, the muscles must work harder in cases of excessive body weight. However, research has shown that unless an exercise programme, designed specifically to improve muscle capacity is undertaken, the body muscles retain a size and strength appropriate for the ideal body weight of the subject, rather than remodelling to accommodate excess weight.

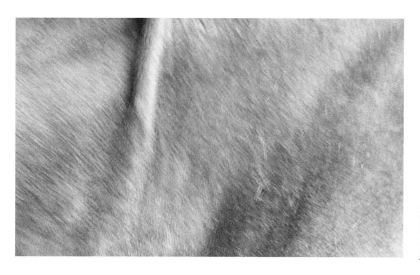

Dehydration – the skin should not remain as a raised fold.

112

A horse in a prepared box with a rug to keep the hindquarters warm while the neck and shoulders are massaged.

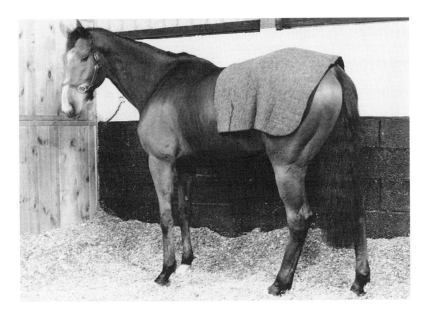

A similar response has not been recorded in the horse. However, it can be stated that very fat horses are not capable of sustained strenuous activity and a great deal of effort is required to reduce body weight in order to avoid musculo-skeletal breakdown. This would suggest that the muscles of a horse, in common with man, do not build to accommodate for body-induced weight overload.

MAINTENANCE MASSAGE (SWEDISH)

Horse Massage

As previously described the horse is caught, restrained, and the box made ready before the masseur begins to work. A Glentona half rug is very useful in cold weather and easier to work with than a full, heavy rug. Easily laundered, several

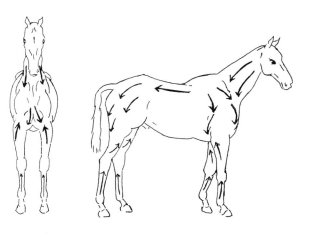

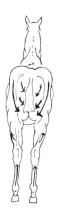

Directions for Swedish Massage.

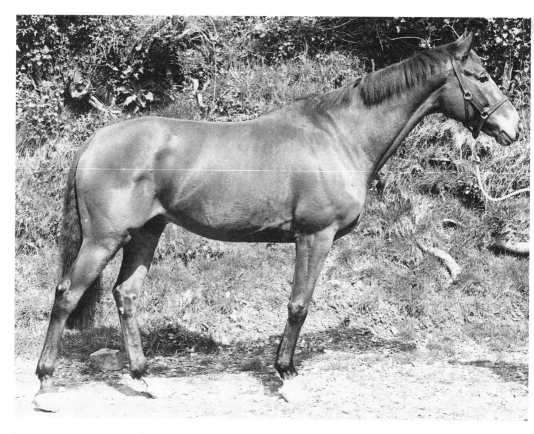

The contour of the muscles can be identified on a conditioned horse.

may be carried from yard to yard, to ensure a clean one is available for each horse – they are equally useful for rider massage. Allow one hour for a full Swedish massage.

The masseur must decide whether to work an entire side or to quarter the horse, finishing one area before moving to another. For those not familiar with the term, to 'quarter' a horse means to mentally divide the body into four equal parts or quarters – head to mid back/loins including the front leg, loins to tail including the hind leg, on the near and off sides.

If quartering, it is probably sensible to work the whole front of the animal, massaging the neck, shoulder and front leg of one side, then moving under the neck to the opposite side, before working each hindquarter individually. To work by quartering is not always suitable for techniques other than Swedish massage.

The contour of the muscles can be identified on a conditioned horse. A quick visual inspection should be followed by an introductory neck rub and then an invitation to the horse to smell the masseur's hands in an 'I am a friend, do not panic' introduction. When the horse has accepted the presence of the masseur, the entire body should be assessed to quantify the general 'feel' of the horse. The hands should pass lightly over the body surface

114

sensing the texture of the coat, locating anatomical landmarks and registering areas of tension, heat, excessive cold or unnatural contour. The masseur should be positioned in such a way as to be able to watch the head and 'read' the horse by observing its ears, eyes, lower lips and tail. When massaging, reading the body language of the horse should be as automatic as glancing in the rear mirror when driving.

The hands can be used flat with fingers spread or closed, one hand may reinforce the other, fingers can be cupped or clenched into fists. The fingers may be used individually or as a group. The thumbs, used singly or as a pair, can work with the fingers or deliver deep pressure.

The ability to seamlessly change with no break in rhythm the position or shape of the hands and fingers and to move smoothly from one technique to another under the wide range of conditions and circumstances, reflects the art of the good masseur.

Neck and Shoulders

The masseur should be positioned near the shoulder, but at a sufficient distance from the horse to allow the use of body weight. The feet should be apart to maintain balance.

The massage starts with the use of lightly applied effleurage. Swedish massage techniques all start distally with the masseur working towards the main venous collection points, the armpits and groin. The hands are first placed on the neck just behind the poll, the strokes can be either double or single-handed. The neck and shoulders are worked in a manner that ensures continuous, rhythmic, overlapping strokes directed towards the centre of the body along the path of the venous blood flow.

Work continues downward, covering the whole side and working slowly over the full expanse of the neck. It is better, particularly in the case of long-necked horses, to use a series of short strokes rather than attempting to cover the area from poll to wither with one long stroke. The hands should progress slowly down the neck towards the front of the shoulder, not forgetting the area from the base of the neck to between the front legs. After finishing the side of the neck and front of the chest, the hands should glide on to reach the shoulder area.

(Note: It is very easy to forget to massage the important musculature of the full neck expanse when giving massage working only along the top line.)

The shoulder is massaged starting from the withers, the hands moving down and forward in front of the spine of the scapula, towards the point of the elbow when massaging the area behind the spine of the shoulder bone. Light contact should be maintained by one or both hands even when changing from one area to another: lifting the hands with subsequent loss of contact immediately reduces any relaxation achieved.

Once the horse begins to relax, pressure over the musculature can be increased to manipulate deeper-sited muscles. Compression techniques follow effleurage – these are worked in a similar direction, but the masseur changes hand usage to suit the area being worked. For example, compression is best delivered by using the fingertips around the poll but the whole hand is used between the forelimbs.

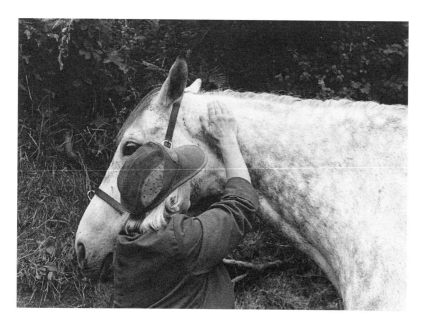

Neck massage – start at the poll using the second hand to support the far side of the neck.

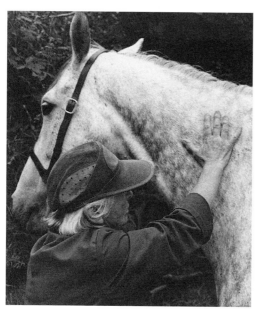

The neck – effleurage can be single-handed, the second hand supporting the opposite side of the neck.

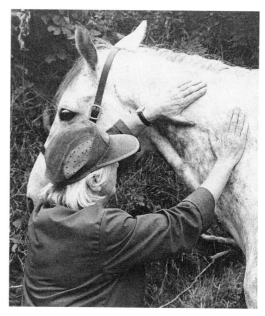

Effleurage can be double-handed.

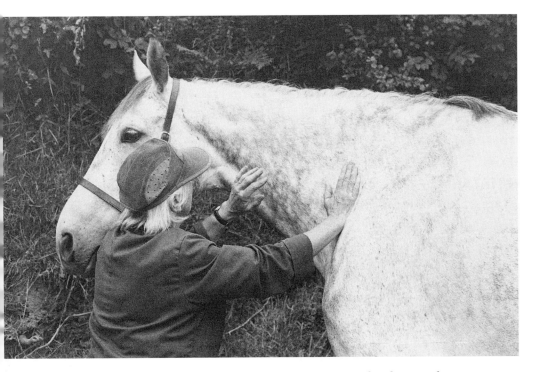

The neck. In double-handed effleurage, as one hand completes a stroke, the second is being repositioned to ensure continuous contact.

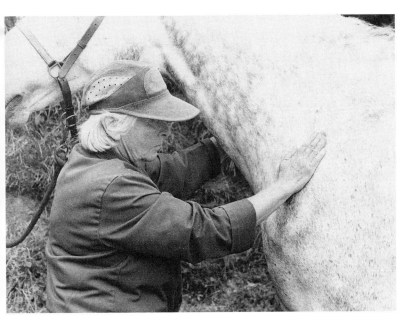

Left and overleaf:
The hands continue to work on the base of the neck.

117

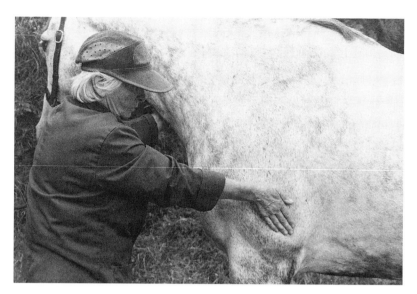

The left hand is working the pectoral muscles. The right hand remains in contact, holding the withers.

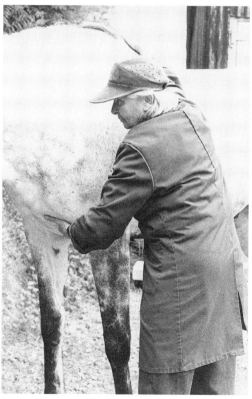

Working down towards the point of the elbow.

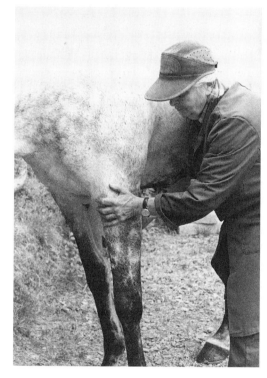

Swedish massage has little effect on a weight-bearing limb, although point stimulation can be successfully executed.

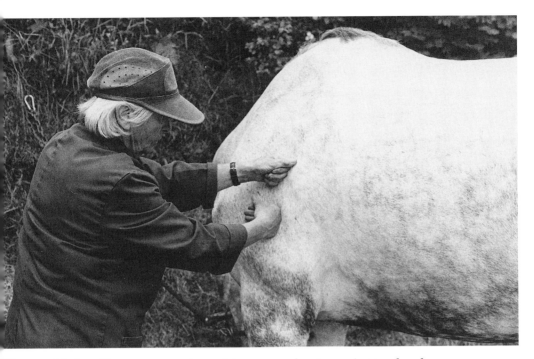

Above and below: *Deeper compression, petrissage, can be given using two hands working alternately, or with one hand reinforced by the second. The technique is executed by pressing in over a relaxed muscle, twisting slightly when deep into the muscle, then bringing the hand or hands to the surface using a small scoop-type action. The hand or hands are moved lightly over the surface to be repositioned for the next compression. A common mistake is to overwork an area causing deep, unwanted bruising.*

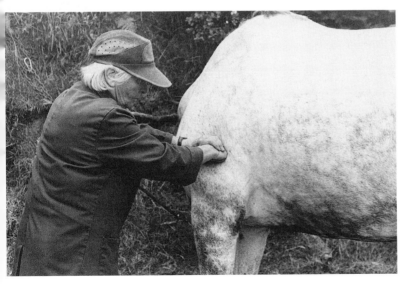

119

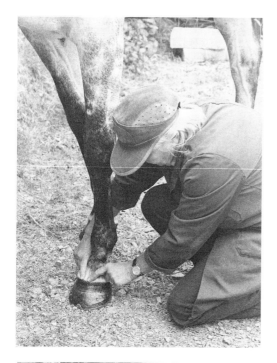

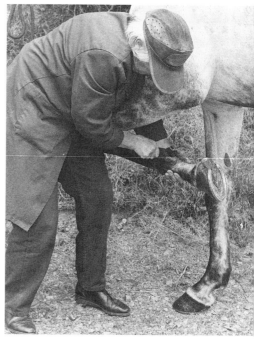

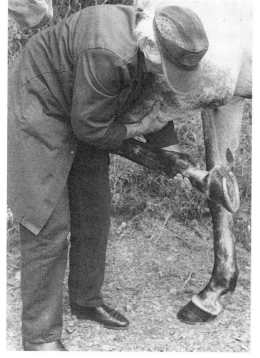

Top left: *The coronet and bulbs of the heels are massaged with the foot on the ground. Circular compression is applied by the fingertips to the coronet, whilst the thumbs press down on the bulbs of the heels.*

Top right: *The leg is picked up, the horse's knee rests on the thigh of the masseur and the shoulder of the horse is pressed against the shoulder of the masseur. With the fetlock held in mid position to avoid proprioceptive input the horse will relax. The tendons are worked between finger and thumb from fetlock to knee.*

Left: *The forearm is worked from knee to elbow using the palm of the operating hand to compress the tissues against the back of the underlying bone. Due to hair lie effleurage cannot be used. The medial side of the forearm can also be worked in this position. The masseur must ensure they bend at hips and knees to avoid back strain.*

Forelimb

Due to the stay system required to maintain stability, the limb musculature always exhibits considerable postural tone. The major muscle bulk lies at the back of the forearm, the extensor muscle is merely a flat expanse with virtually no mass suitable for massage.

While the coronet and heel bulbs are worked with the foot on the ground, the leg should be supported in flexion to ensure effective massage of both the tendons and the muscles of the forearm.

Effleurage cannot be used comfortably due to hair lie so local compression is used, working up the limb towards the axilla. The tendons are massaged with circular compression applied between finger and thumb, the forearm by compression using the palm.

Note: Friction to a tendon is best given with the horse standing, not with the limb in flexion.

Back

If the horse is very tall it may be necessary for the masseur to use a box to stand on. If this is the case, a helper should always be present or near at hand even if the horse is used to such a device – never forget that safety is the primary consideration.

Swedish massage is directed only at the muscles supporting the back and not extended to work over the ribs. The back is worked directionally from withers to lumbar sacral junction. As with the neck, effleurage for relaxation is followed by local compression. The most effective compression technique is to clump the

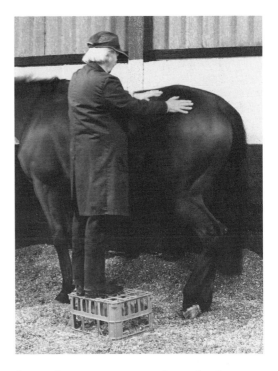

It may be necessary to stand on a box to achieve the correct working height to massage the back.

fingertips together and describe continuous, small circles from behind the withers to the quarter mass.

The muscle mass extends laterally from the posterior superior spines, ending where the ribs curl downward. The mass is deepest adjacent to the posterior superior spines, reducing laterally towards the outer edge of the cage formed by the ribs.

The back musculature is in constant tone both to resist gravity and to ensure stability of the vertebral column. Some relaxation will result if the horse can be persuaded to rest the hind limb of the side of the body being worked.

It is impossible to massage the back without influencing zones and meridians.

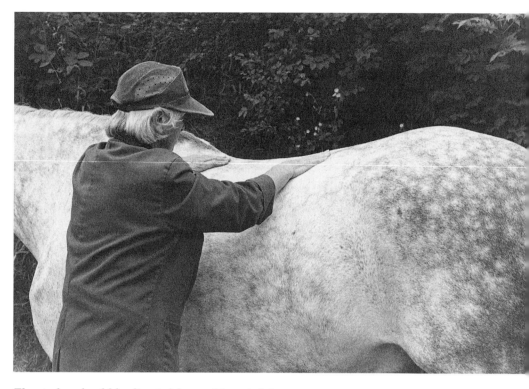

The strokes should be directed from withers to loins.

Hindquarters

The masseur must find a position that is safe, practical and from where the horse's body language may be observed, not only looking at the head but also watching the tail. Tails can be very expressive – relaxed, all is well; clamped or swished, watch out!

The massage commences with *effleurage*, using shorter strokes than for the neck or back. The hind quarter mass is worked towards but not into the groin. The routine is best executed if the strokes begin just in front of the loins and sweep towards the tail root with each ensuing stroke fanning back and down from the loins towards the hamstring muscle group. The hamstrings can be worked from the tail root down towards the groin.

Compression techniques require considerable pressure to be effective, up to 14lb (6.3kg) of thrust is required. This best applied with a lightly clenched fist.

Note: The hamstrings are the only muscle group in the horse where wringing can be successfully used.

Opposite top: *It may be necessary to stand on a box to achieve a working height for massaging the hindquarters. Strokes are performed from loins towards the tail root and on downwards covering the whole muscle mass while avoiding the tuber coccae (point of hip).*

122

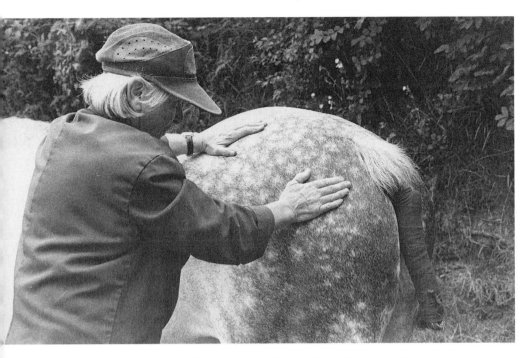

When massaging the hind quarters the strokes are directed from loins to tail root and on downward, covering the whole muscle mass while avoiding the tuber coccae.

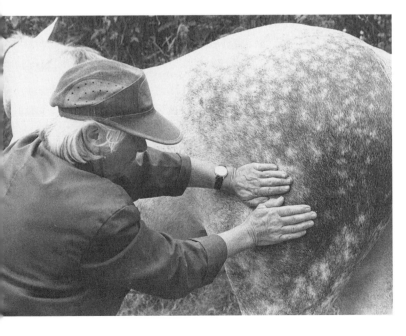

The upper hand is covering the greater trocanter, the lower hand is operative.

123

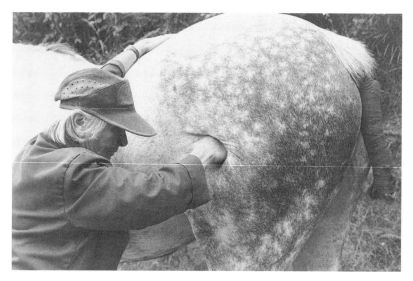

Really deep compression is required to influence the major muscle groups of the hind leg.

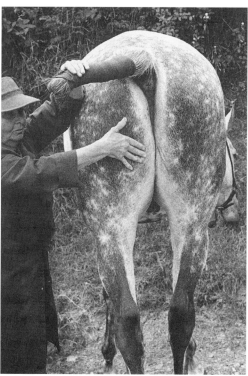

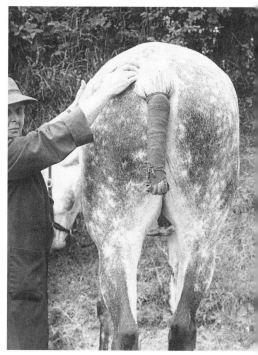

The hamstrings are worked down and in towards the groin. The tail is held to the side to demonstrate the muscles.

Local compression to biceps femoris. The muscle originates on the lateral aspect of the sacrum and is often uncomfortable following demanding exercise involving the hind limbs.

124

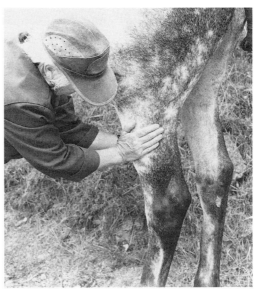

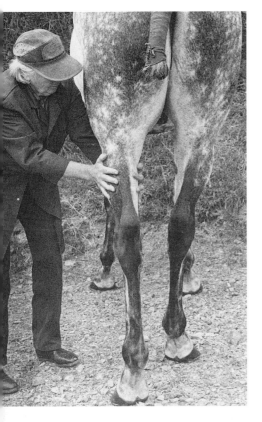

Above and left: *Hand position to influence the second thigh or gaskin. The hands can be worked as a pair from hock to thigh using an alternating upward circling movement. The horse is not resting the leg so massage would be ineffective. Point stimulation is given with the leg in a weight-bearing position.*

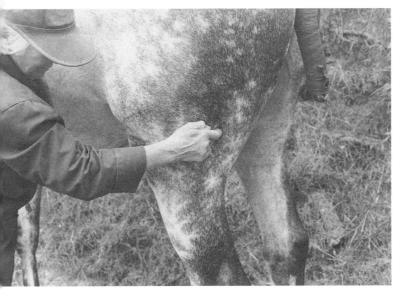

Left: *The fingers are used in this way to influence trigger points, stress points, motor points or ashi points.*

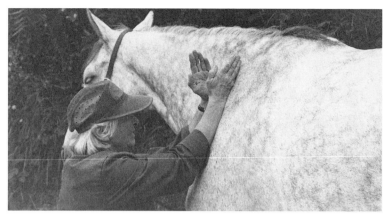

Left, above and below:
*Following a full body
massage with hacking
and clapping.*

Hacking.

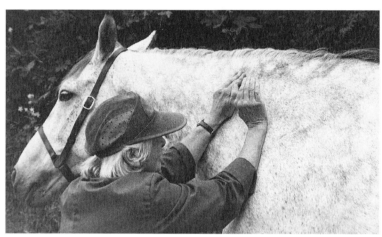

*Clapping. Correct – the
hands are cupped.*

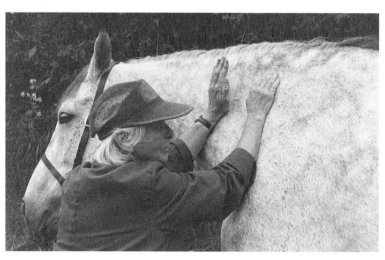

*Clapping. Incorrect –
if the hands are not
cupped a slap will
result.*

Hind Limb

As with the forelimb, postural tone throughout the stay system reduces the masseur's ability to be fully effective. The horse should be taught to rest the hind leg and remain thus during hindquarter and hind limb massage. Effleurage cannot be used comfortably due to hair lie, and local compression is the best alternative.

The coronet and heel bulb are worked with the foot flat, then the horse is asked to rest the limb. The tendons are worked between fingers and thumb; the second thigh muscles are gently compressed inward against the underlying bone.

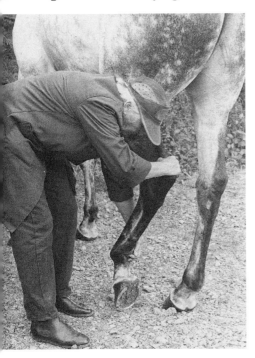

Massage of the whole hindquarter mass and hind leg is much more effective if the horse can be persuaded to rest the hind leg during massage. It often takes two to three sessions before this becomes an automatic response on the part of the horse.

MASSAGE FOR THE RIDER

In an ideal world the subject should begin the massage session lying face down, relaxed and warm, on a couch of a height that enables the masseur to work without excessive back strain. Normally the upper back and neck are worked first, followed by the low back, then the backs and sides of each leg. The arms, each supported in turn by a pillow, are worked when the subject turns to lie face up. Apart from the target area, the body should be covered both for warmth, relaxation and modesty.

At competition, necessity can prove to be the mother of invention. In an ideal situation, massage is given with the subject stripped. However, working with riders in a yard or at a competition often makes this impossible. It is often necessary to work through clothes, making the use of effleurage impossible and necessitating a suitable adaptation of most other techniques. Relaxation of the target area is essential and ingenuity will usually create some method of achieving this. For example, it is perfectly possible for the masseur to kneel down and use the ground as a base. However, a folding couch, a towel and at least one pillow should be routine equipment. The venue for massage is governed by circumstances, but the subject, as already stated, should be lying down and as warm, relaxed and comfortably supported as possible. If there is one essential factor required in the equine masseur it is responsible versatility, for those requiring help are certainly not lying relaxed in a cosy treatment scenario, but more often are cold, covered in mud and irritable.

As hip flexibility is essential for all who ride, massage should be followed by

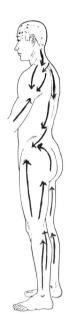
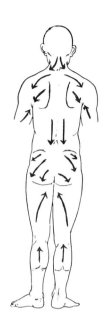
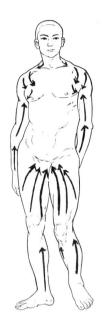

*Stroke direction –
Swedish massage.*

hip stretching. Prolonged stretching is not necessary, stretching twice quite adequate.

Neck

The neck is worked from the base of the skull down and out over the top and back of the shoulders, then towards the axilla.

Back

From the base of the neck, the back is worked down to the lumbar area then out and forward towards the groin.

Limbs

Each arm is worked from hand to axilla and each leg from foot to groin.

Each sport stresses particular areas; riding is no exception. In riders, unless extenuating factors such as a fall have occurred, in which case each circumstance must be considered and addressed appropriately, the following areas of stress are common to all.

Base of the Neck to the Point of the Shoulder

The muscles of this area stabilize the shoulder joint, allowing the arms to hold the reins in the various positions required by individual disciplines. The muscles must also resist the forward stress exerted at the shoulder joint in a horse that pulls. All those involved in driving horses stress these muscles.

The design of the shoulder joint makes it entirely dependent upon the muscles and ligaments for stability and

128

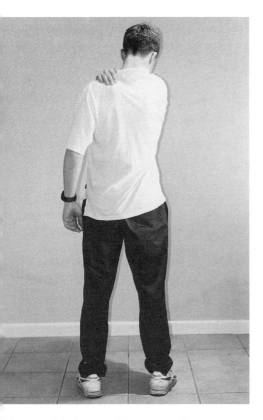

Massage for the muscles running from the base of the neck to the point of the shoulder using small circular compressions.

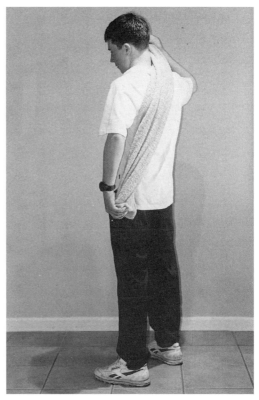

Using a towel to massage both mid and upper back.

function, and dislocation is a common rider injury.

Massage   Use effleurage to relax. Follow with finger compression.

Self-help   Cross an arm over the front of the chest, placing the fingers over the area described and work outward from the base of the neck to the shoulder, using the fingers to perform a series of small, circular movements.

Low Back

A common area of discomfort is the central area from the bottom of the ribs down over the back. The area is covered by a diamond-shaped sheet of fascia into which the long muscles of the back intertwine from above and those of the buttocks blend from below. The deep muscles' functioning to support the lumbar vertebrae and ensure stability at the lumbar sacral junction, are sited below this fascia lying immediately adjacent to the lumbar vertebrae.

As in the horse, there are muscles inside the pelvis, originating from the front and sides of the vertebrae then running

129

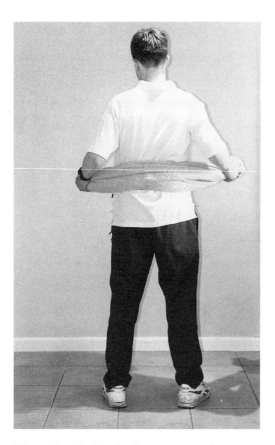

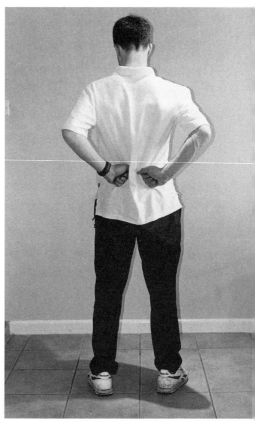

Massaging the low back using a towel.

The rider is massaging the low back or lumbar area using the fists to perform a bilateral, circular, compressive technique.

forward and downward to attach near the groin on the front of the pubic bone. Disruption to the natural angle of the lumbar spine, particularly when a rider rearranges the angle of the spine to change their seat, rather than repositioning at the hips, stresses these internal muscles and often reflects pain into the groin.

Massage   Effleurage, working out from the centre of the back towards the groin. Compression, using the fingers, works through the fascia to affect the small multipennate muscles.

Self-help   Treat by rubbing – place a towel over the area and pull back and forth. Pummelling with clenched fists, gently at first then gradually building up force increases local circulation.

Buttocks and Sacroiliac Area

Strain of the sacroiliac joint is the cause of more discomfort in the general populace

130

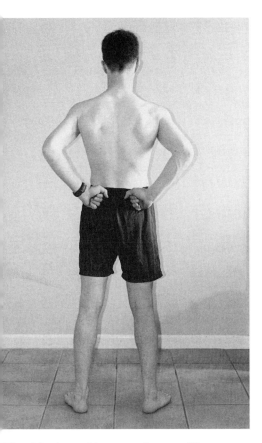

The rider is working over the sacroiliac joints. These joints are stressed along with the lumbar spine when the pelvic angle is incorrectly rearranged. As there is little muscle in the area, gentle banging with the clenched fists can be used to improve local circulation.

than strain in almost any other joint. The joint acts as a shock absorber rather than as a true joint – active movement is neither catered for nor possible. For support, the joint relies upon a complex ligament plexus rather than muscle alone.

The lumbar sacral junction, the sacroiliac joints and the hip joints all interact together, relying each upon the other for

an appropriate, calculated range of motion during activity. Reduced hip mobility stresses this interaction and forces the sacroiliac joints and the lumbar sacral junction to reposition, often resulting in pain.

In the early stages this pain may be locally perceived but due to the phenomenon of referred pain, discomfort can be experienced anywhere throughout the associated limb dermatome. Leg pain is often wrongly attributed to disc protrusion. Sacroiliac pain usually hurts in bed, making getting up difficult, but improves when the subject becomes active; disc pain usually gets worse with activity, reducing in bed or when the subject lies flat.

Massage   If pain will allow, local friction of the ligaments lying over the back of the joint.

Self-help   Locate the painful spot over the irritable joint and rub it hard using stress or *ashi* point type massage.

Massage of the buttock muscles reduces spasm secondary to pain from the sacroiliac joints and is required to prepare the muscles for stretching. Use effleurage followed by compression, working from the centre towards the groin following a similar fan pattern to that adopted for the gluteal mass of the horse.

The Thighs and Lower Leg

The thigh muscles, in particular those lying over the front of the thigh, the quadriceps, are continually active in the rider, particularly at trot when

131

together with the buttock muscles they control rider movement in the hip and knee joints.

The thrust generated by the hind-quarter muscles of the horse should push the rider effortlessly out of the saddle. The thigh and buttock muscles then work eccentrically to lower the rider back into the saddle – a very strenuous muscle activity.

The adductor muscles hold the thighs against the saddle. The effort created within these muscles increases their functional power to a degree that hip mobility is eventually reduced. In order to retain hip mobility, it is essential that the rider should learn correct adductor stretching. The adductors are best influenced by active stretching following a full leg massage. If torn, local friction is appropriate.

The muscles running down the outer side of the lower leg, the perenei, are involved in positioning the heel for application of the 'aids'.

Massage   Thigh: effleurage, wringing and compression.

Self-help Position by sitting with the knees bent and muscles relaxed. Effleurage, working from the knee towards the groin using a spread palm. Follow by holding the muscle mass between fingers and thumb, lifting away, squeezing and releasing.

Lower leg: effleurage and local compression.

Still sitting, lean forward and work the muscles on the outer side of the lower leg from ankle to knee using the finger-tips.

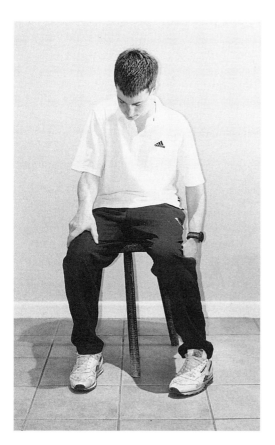

Massaging the quadriceps muscles by holding the muscle mass between fingers and thumbs.

AREAS OF FATIGUE ASSOCIATED WITH VARIOUS DISCIPLINES

If there is no time for a full body massage, concentrate on the areas suggested for each discipline preferably before and after activity. The techniques suggested are based on those used in Swedish massage routines rather than the use of stress or *ashi* points.

Riding for Recreation

Horse

A number of horses return from a ride with mild discomfort in their back. They have not injured themselves but unaccustomed activity, inadequate muscle preparation and possibly a poorly fitting saddle have resulted in muscular discomfort.

The natural way for a horse to relieve an aching back is to roll. However, rolling in a box causes endless problems, horses often becoming cast and then injuring themselves in their violent efforts to get up on to their feet. In former times, large yards were equipped with sand rolls and at the conclusion of exercise, after being unsaddled, all horses were taken to the sand area and encouraged to roll. Allowed

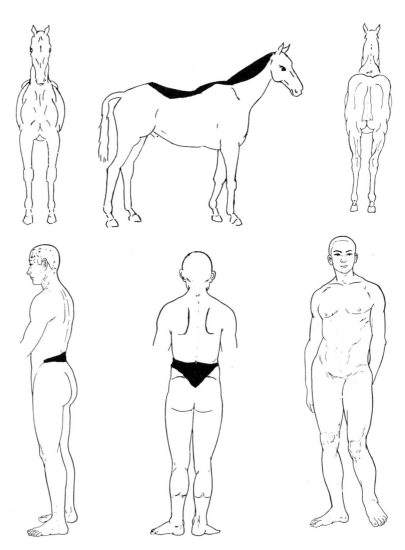

Recreational riding – stress areas.

this opportunity, horses rarely rolled in their boxes.

If the horse has enough space to allow it to roll and turn right over, any minor back derangement sustained during exercise will rectify naturally because postural tone throughout the back is reduced significantly, allowing minor movements between adjoining vertebrae and their associated facet joints to occur. As any adjoining anatomical surfaces will always return to their anatomical normal given the chance to do so, there is a very strong case for allowing horses to roll to avoid or rectify minor back problems.

Massage	The back from mid neck to the hindquarter mass, paying particular attention to the loins.
Strokes	Effleurage, compression, hacking, clapping.

Rider

Low-back discomfort is not confined to the horse.

Massage	Low back.
Strokes	Effleurage, compression.
Self-help	Towel massage the low back and pummel gently. Stretch adductors and possibly flex hips.

Dressage

Horse

The discipline is very exhausting both mentally and physically. Few horses, other than those trained in the European classical schools, are given sufficient time to prepare the muscles for dressage as this process can take years.

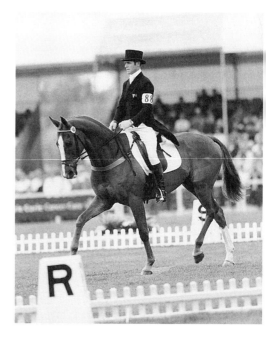

An outline must be maintained.

To perform a balanced circle is, for an animal that would never attempt such a feat in a natural state, an immensely difficult task. It takes months to prepare the muscles, to learn balanced co-ordination of all four limbs, and to programme the brain to automatically produce the required pattern of movement co-ordination on command.

In dressage, the outline required necessitates static muscle work for the axial skeleton. Much of the limb activity requires middle-range muscle work and the stresses to stifle and hock during advanced work are almost incalculable.

Massage	The poll, working down to the angle of the jaw to include the cheek muscles. Mid neck to behind the withers.

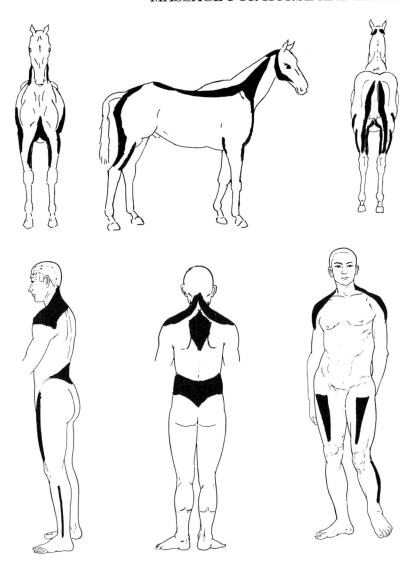

Dressage – stress areas.

Forearm and adductor muscles.
Loins.
Hamstring.
Second thigh and adductor muscles.

Strokes Effleurage, finger compression, wringing (hamstrings).

Rider

The rider with immobile hips will have the greatest difficulty in riding a good test.

Massage Upper back, shoulders and base of neck.
Low back.
Front of the thighs.
Outer side of the lower leg.

135

	Active hip stretching if the rider is relaxed and warm.
Strokes	Effleurage, kneading, local compression using fingertips.
Self-help	Towel-massage low back and across shoulders.

Endurance

Horse

This discipline continues to become more demanding, the time factor necessitating a considerable amount of trotting over very varied terrain. To avoid foot bruises, the wearing of protective sole pads has become commonplace. However, care should be taken as they undoubtedly result in slippage and damaged muscles if the ground is wet and rock strewn. At competition, the masseur should assess the course in the light of their experience of the client's training methods and home terrain, and adapt the massage routine to accommodate. For example, horses trained on flat land cannot cope easily with hills, those trained on good going will not be prepared for deep going.

Massage	The back from withers to loins.
	Shoulder muscles.
	Hamstrings, second thigh.
Strokes	Effleurage, gentle hacking and clapping.

Other strokes can be incorporated but the horse may well resent deep compressions. As the object is to relax the animal so that it will drink and feed, to cause pain and anxiety is counter-productive.

Massaging with cold towels will help reduce the body temperature and contribute to reducing the heart rate at veterinary checks.

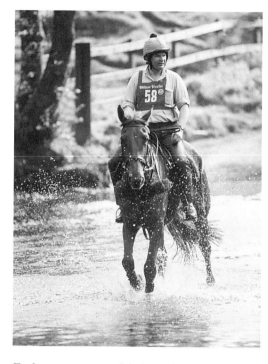

Endurance – general fatigue if not conditioned.

Rider

Riders who dismount and run, particularly downhill, will be helped by a leg massage. Back and neck discomfort are usually caused by the saddle type used. The 'Western' allows an easy seat with little or no rider discomfort reported. 'Borrowed' saddles or a new design not properly broken in, need to be assessed and their stress points identified.

Most endurance riders have learnt to alter leather length during the ride so lessening fatigue by changing muscle recruitment.

Massage	Low back.
	Front and inside of thigh.
	Calf muscles.

Endurance – stress areas.

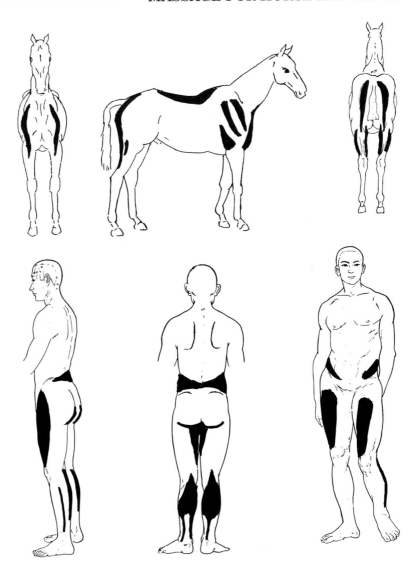

| Stroke | Effleurage. |
| Self-help | Rub thigh and calf muscles, shaking to relax. |

Cross-Country Events

Horse

Hunter trials, team chasing, and eventing all require a series of obstacles to be jumped while galloping across tracts of natural land.

Massage   A general body massage (use ice massage for bruised areas).

Note: Falls should be assessed by a veterinary surgeon prior to any form of massage.

137

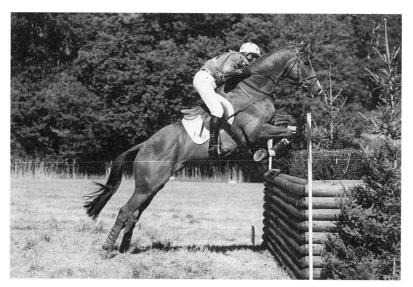

*Cross-country –
hind limb thrust
prior to tak-eoff.*

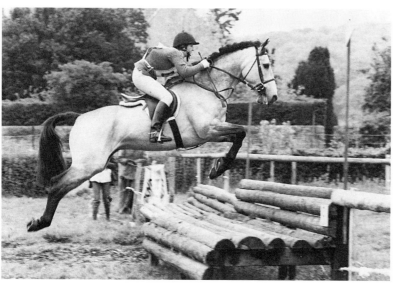

*Hunter trials – note
the limb angles, as
they act as levers.*

Rider

Due to the respiratory confines of modern body protectors, many event riders are generally exhausted and probably more dehydrated than they realize after the road, track and steeplechase sections on cross-country day.

Do not massage unless satisfied that the discomfort described is genuine muscular fatigue, not that caused by dehydration or anoxia.

Low-back fatigue is common to all areas, but the shoulders, mid back and limbs are usually only painful following a

138

Cross-country events – stress areas.

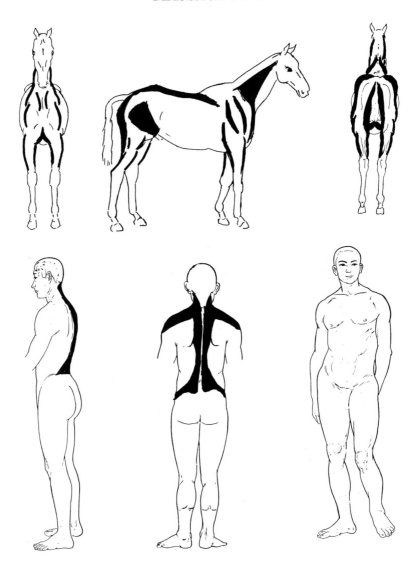

horse error which has caught the rider off balance.

Massage   Full back massage if possible, other areas as appropriate.

Strokes   Effleurage, local compression.

Self-help   Rehydrate, relax. During competition (eventing, point-to-point) loosen body protector if very restrictive and try to take several easy breaths to reduce possible oxygen deficit.

For the three-day event rider, a full body massage on the morning before the show jumping will improve flexibility.

139

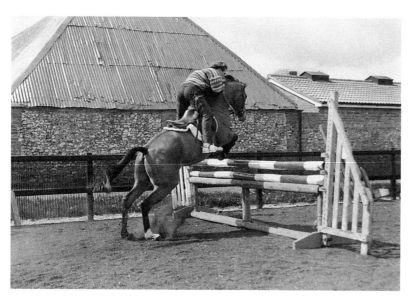

Show-jumping take-off – note the pastern angle in both hind legs.

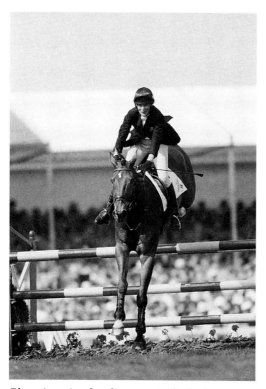

Show jumping landing – note the body weight will land through the near fore.

Show Jumping

Horse
Show jumping demands spurts of high-density energy. The inside hind leg is subjected to severe stress on turns when jumping against the clock. Bruising is common when poles are knocked. Horses may slip badly – the huge effort to rebalance may often lead to a torque strain to the back.

Massage   General body massage before and after competition. Locating tension areas following a bad round or practice-ring incident is important, choose the technique appropriate for the individual horse to achieve general muscle relaxation. (It is for this reason that masseurs must know the horses with which they are expected to work at competition.)

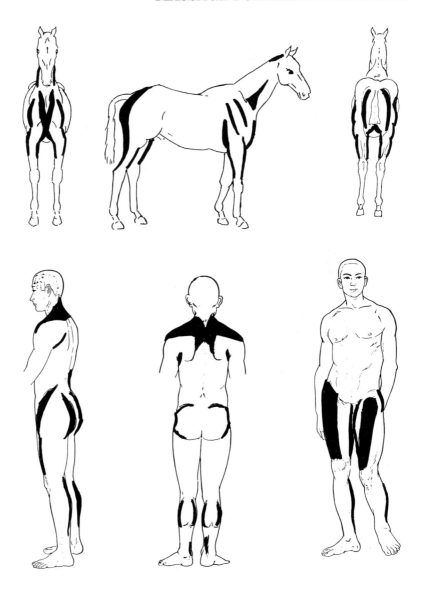

Show jumping – stress areas.

Ice massage may be required in cases of severe bruising.

Rider

The hips and knees are continually in action as the rider rearranges the body to take weight off the horse's back.

Massage	Shoulders, low back, hips.
Strokes	Effleurage, compression.
Self-help	Towel or rub low back, rub fronts of thighs.

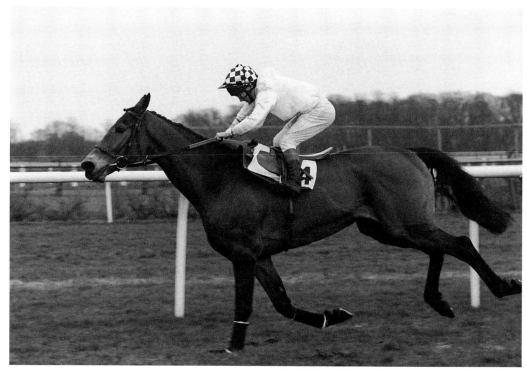

Flat racing – breaking from the starting stalls damages the hindquarters. The jockey rides on his knees.

Flat Racing

Horse
Breaking from the stalls causes stress to the musculature of the hind quarters, particularly the hamstring muscles. Sacroiliac joint strain is also common.

Massage	Loins, hindquarter mass, hamstring group. Elbow and shoulder.
Strokes	Effleurage, compression, wringing.

Jockey
The flat-race jockey is never in the saddle – standing in the irons with knees and hips taking the full strain, the muscles often have to work in a static manner until forced into action as the jockey rides a finish.

The muscles of flat jockeys feel as though they are made of steel wires. Massage with care as there is no spare flesh, and always consider the possibility of dehydration due to diuretics and excessive sauna usage.

Massage	Upper back, low back, thigh and calf muscles.
Strokes	Effleurage, gentle compression.
Self-help	Rarely considered useful – they prefer to be massaged professionally.

*Flat racing –
stress areas.*

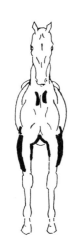
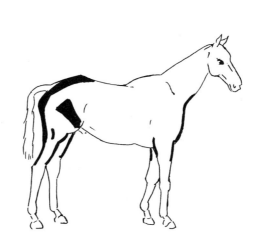
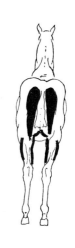

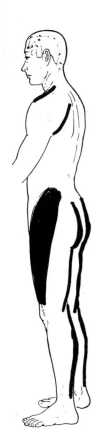
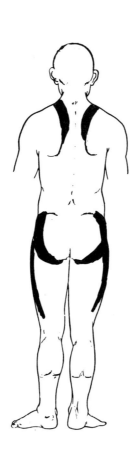
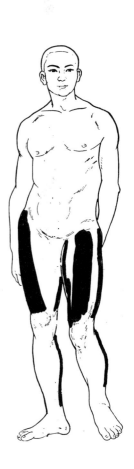

143

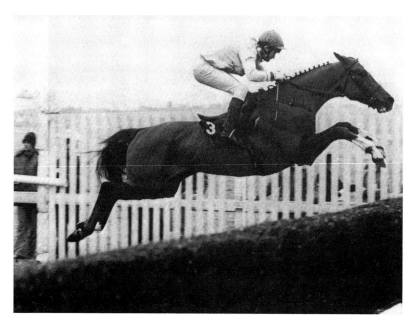

National Hunt Horse. Note the loose rein, the jockey balancing over the centre of gravity.

National Hunt

Horse

A number of horses become very excited when they arrive at a racecourse. Experience has shown that massage after arrival relaxes a stressed animal and improves performance results.

National Hunt horses are often said to pull out stiff on the day following a race. Massage, if hydration levels are normal, reduces the post-race recovery period and enables horses to return rapidly to their normal training routine.

Falls should be reported to the masseur who should try to watch it on the race video as the angle, speed and type of fall helps pinpoint stressed or bruised areas.

Massage	Full body massage. Selection of the appropriate technique depends on the area of trauma.

Jockey

The National Hunt jockey rides with a number of chronic minor injuries as they fall, on average, once in every seven rides. The neck and shoulders are commonly stressed.

The racing industry is the only equine discipline with strict rules regarding falls and jockey injury. All jockeys carry an injury book and have to be examined by a doctor appointed by the racing authorities before they are allowed to ride again following any fall that has resulted in an entry in their book.

Always make certain jockeys are not making light of their problems. Do not massage if there is any uncertainty about this or if there is a possibility of concussion.

Massage	Neck and shoulders, low back.
Strokes	Effleurage, compression.
Self-help	Towel-massage shoulders and low back.

144

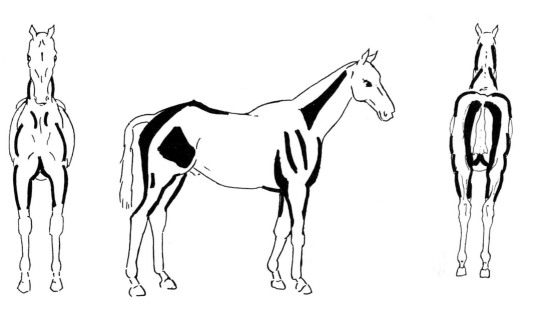

National Hunt – stress areas.

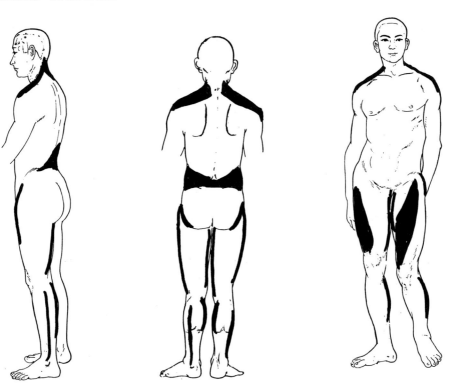

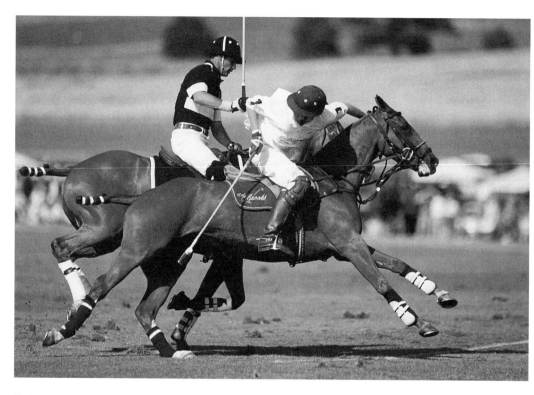

Polo.

Polo

Horse

The game requires acceleration, deceleration, turns, and extreme efforts of balance.

Massage	Neck, loins, hamstrings, abductor and adductor muscles.
Strokes	Effleurage, compression.

Rider
Bruising from being hit by a ball or another player's stick is common.

Massage	Low back and shoulders.
Strokes	Effleurage, compression.
Self-help	Towel-massage shoulders, rub low back, adductor stretch.

Driving

Horse

The driven horse leans into a collar or breast harness to pull and sits on the breeching to help brake. The masseur should be familiar with the capabilities and performance of each horse if working with a team. If one horse does not work as it should, added stress will be transferred to the second horse of a pair. In a team of four, the line of pull will angle incorrectly if one horse is being 'carried' by the others.

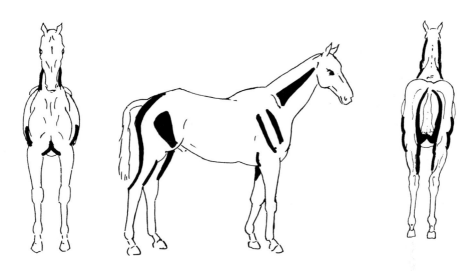

Polo – stress areas.

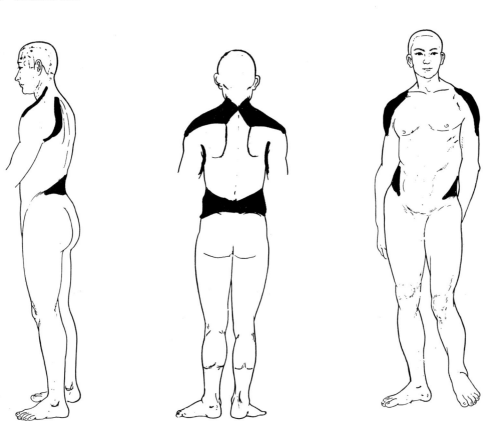

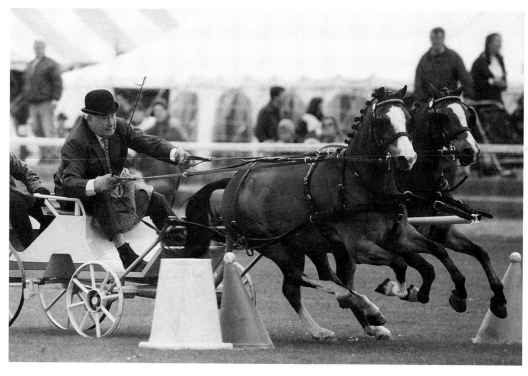

Driving.

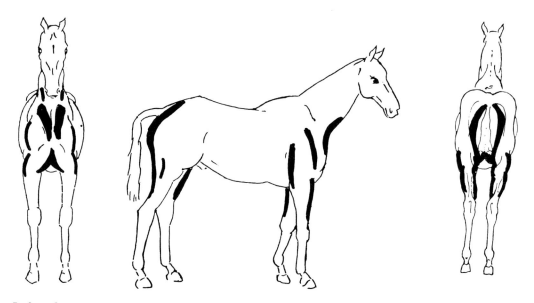

Left and opposite: *Driving – stress areas.*

148

Massage   Lower area of the neck,
           hamstrings, abductors and
           adductors.
Strokes   Effleurage, compression,
           wringing.

Driver
The severity of stress varies upon the type
of driving competition and the number of
horses being driven.

Massage   Shoulders and arms, low
           back, thighs, calves.
Strokes   Effleurage, compression,
           wringing.
Self-help Towel-massage shoulders and
           low back. Rub fronts of thighs
           and calf muscles.

STRESS POINTS RELATED TO BODY AREA DYSFUNCTION IN THE HORSE

It must be clearly understood that the
following list, which associates stress
points located in named muscles to bio-
mechanical dysfunction, does not mean
that stimulation of the suggested stress
points will necessarily resolve the
problem. For example, rigidity on one rein
may be tooth related – most problems are
multi-factorial.

Therapy is easy – it is identifying the
cause of a problem that presents the
challenge!

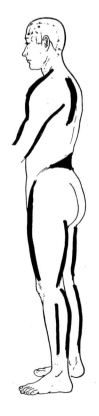
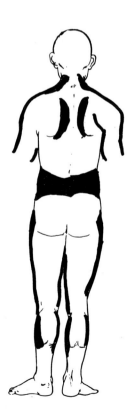
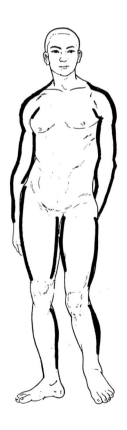

149

The Neck

Signs of dysfunction	*Muscle in which stress point is located*
Discomfort/resistance to side flexion.	Rectus capitis ventralis
Resistance to neck flexion, tries to stretch down.	Splenius Cervicus
Continual high head carriage, resistance to flexion, inability to lift under the rider.	Brachiocephalic
Rigidity on one or other rein.	Omohyoid and sternohyoid
Shortening of forelimb stride.	Scalene and/or serratus cervicis

Shoulder area

Incorrect scapula action associated with shortening of stride and possibly increase in knee flexion.	Supra and/or infraspinatus
Reacts to tightening the girth.	Caudal fibres trapezius
Shortens stride, reluctance going downhill.	
Reluctance to move laterally on one rein.	Descending pectoral of the limb

The Back

Reluctance to lift back, goes hollow.	Caudal fibres trapezius
Stiff back, unable to bascule.	Longissimus dorsi (usually several areas of the muscle are affected)

The Hindquarters

Cold back.	Caudal fibres of longissimus
Restricted hind leg action.	Superficial gluteal
Scuffs hind toe, hock screws.	Biceps femoris
Poor lateral movement of one hind.	Vastus lateralis of the limb the horse is reluctant/unable to move laterally
Backs up unevenly, shortened forward stride.	Gastrocnemius
Prefers one lead, may go disunited of asked to change leads.	Vastus lateralis

Swedish and Stress Point massage are directed primarily at enhancement of normal muscle function. CTM and Bowen are directed primarily at recovery following injury. Acupressure, Tteam and Shiatsu are all methods of influencing the behaviour of the total body. Swedish and Stress Point Massage necessitates a learning curve associated with the musculo-skeletal system only, and while it is undeniable that each methodology marginally overlaps the other and none can be reliably stated to achieve a specific isolated effect, CTM, Bowen, Tteam, Shiatsu and certainly Acupressure should only be practiced after adequate, in-depth training.

Appendix I ————————————

Possible Links Between Superficial Points and Organs in the Horse (Giniaux, 1996 *see* Bibliography)

It is important to note that the following has not been scientifically verified.

Level/ dermatome	Disorder	Problem, organic/functional
Occiput	Difficult to ride	Sad/aggressive
	Asymmetric hind leg activity	Behavioural problem
C1	Eyesight problems	Headache, sad, dislikes bright light
C2	Tooth/jaw pain	Throat problems
	Fight rider's hands	Gutteral pouch infection
	Chews incorrectly	
C5	Hangs one-sided	Pituitary, hormonal
C7	Neuralgia	Circulatory disturbance
	Cervico brachical	Front legs. Bone and tendon
	Lame in front	problems
C7/T1		Feeding/digestive problems
		Impairment of stellate ganglia function
T2/T3	Stumbling when ridden	
T4,5,6,	Stiff shoulders	Impaired respiration
Withers	High head carriage	
T8/10	(Not identified)	Heart/lung affected
T12/13	Crib biting	Stomach disorders including ulcers
T14		Chronic myositis
		Liver problems
T15		Spleen problems
T17	Pacing	Glandular problems
		Tendency to colic
		Dry pellet droppings
L1	Stiff behind	Ovarian problems
		Pain in inguinal canal
L2	Pulls off a front shoe	Kidney irritation
L3	Stifle/patella	Small-intestine problems
L6	Stands off fences, low weak heels behind	Bladder problems

Appendix II ———————————

Any person offering massage or an associated therapy should:

- Hold a valid insurance which covers them to work with both horses and humans.
- Have contacted the veterinary surgeon normally used by the owner/rider, or if at competition the senior veterinary officer.
- Report to the doctor whom the person would normally attend if any type of injury occurred.
- Have suitably executed, legally approved, liability forms. Such a form should be signed by any person receiving therapy prior to their first massage, or in the case of a horse by the owner, the rider or a designated person acting with permission of the owner or rider.

The legal requirements for those offering and being paid for integrative or complementary therapies are constantly being changed and updated. For example, it constitutes a legal offence to offer osteopathic adjustment unless on the official register.

The format of sample record forms follow.

Sample Record Sheet

Horses Name . . . .

Breed . . . . .Discipline . . . .

Age/Sex/Colour . . . .

Owner . . . .

Address . . . .

. . . .

. . . . .Code . . . .

Tel . . . . .Fax . . . .

Trainer/Rider . . . .

Address . . . .

. . . .

Tel . . . . .Fax . . . .

Vet . . . .

Address . . . .

. . . .

Tel . . . . .Fax . . . .

History

Blemishes, scars first visit. Pain areas found.

First Assessment   Date . . . . . .

continued overleaf

153

Sample Record Sheet (Rider)

Name ....DOB/Age ....Sex ....

Address ....

....Code ....

Tel ....Fax ....Mob ....

Doctor details ....

....

Doctor contacted .....date ....Report sent ....

Rider discipline ....Experienced/Novice ....

Date first seen ....

History

    NB This should include previous problems, medication, conditions
ie: epilepsy, diabetes.

Type of massage given.

Anatomical Glossary

Abduction Moving outward from the median plane.

Acupoint Specified points on the body relating to the practice of Acupuncture.

Acupressure The stimulation of points using pressure.

Acupuncture The stimulation of points using needles.

Acute A condition having a short, relatively sudden course.

Adhesion Fibrous bands abnormally joining tissues together.

Aids A method of delivering signals from rider to horse.

Appendicular Skeleton The skeletal structures forming the limbs.

Ashi point A painful point in a muscle.

Atrophy Decrease in the size of a muscle or organ resulting from disease or lack of use.

Autonomic Nervous System That part of the nervous system responsible for automatic control of a function, e.g. the heart beat.

Axial Skeleton The vertebral column, the thoracic cage and the pelvis.

Cardiac Pertaining to the heart.

Caudal Toward the tail.

Chi Energy Life force energy considered in Oriental Medicine.

Chronic A condition that persists over a long period with little change or improvement.

Closing Used with acupressure, the stroking technique mirrors effleurage.

Cranial Toward the head.

Connective Tissue The tissue which connects all the various structures of the body, which also acts as a support medium for blood vessels, nerves and nerve endings.

Distal Outward from the centre of a body.

Dorsal Relating to or situated at or close to the back of the body, or to the posterior part of an organ.

Edema (oedema) The presence of abnormally large amounts of fluid between the cells in tissue.

Fascia Sheets of specialist connective tissue forming membranous layers of varied thickness throughout the body mass. Superficial fascia lies immediately below the skin and is contiguous with the deep fascia forming muscle sheaths and surrounding organs.

Fracture A breakage of bone.

Gogli sensors Nerve receptors responding to pressure or stretch.

Haematoma A collection of blood free within tissue that clots and can form a solid swelling.

Insertion The area where a tissue such as muscle, tendon or ligament attaches to bone.

Interossius Between two or more bones.

Intra vertebral Between vertebrae.

Lateral Toward the outside of the body.

Ligaments Connective tissue bands that span joints and join bones.

Lumbar Pertaining to the loins, the part of the back between thorax and pelvis.

Medial Toward the body centre.

Meridian Individual, conceived channels through which the natural energy of the body flows. There are twelve major meridians in all animals (oriental concept).

Motor Point The nerve control centre of a muscle.

Neural Receptor A nerve cell or group of cells programmed to detect changes and respond accordingly.

155

Neurone One of the basic functional units of the nervous system.

Origin The site of muscle attachment that remains relatively fixed as the muscle contracts.

Palpate To feel or perceive through the sensation of touch.

Point The site for acu stimulation.

Proximal Nearer or toward the centre of the body.

Reflex An autonomic or involuntary reaction in response to a sensation or stimulation.

Relaxation Diminution of tension in a muscle

Scar Tissue Tissue laid down following damage to soft tissue.

Spasm Sustained involuntary muscle contraction occuring in response to pain.

Spinous process An upward bone projection from a vertebral body.

Trigger Point A term describing a sensitive point within a muscle which will influence behaviour if stimulated.

Zone A specified area described in Ttouch techniques responsive to stimulation.

Useful Addresses ——

COURSE SOURCES

Beth Course – Bowen
De Mara
Duro Road
Cheltenham
Gloucestershire
GL50 2PD

D'al School of Equine Massage Therapy
672 Matland Street
London
Ontario
N5Y 2V7
Canada

Equine Acupressure Inc.
PO Box 123
Parker
CO 80134
USA

Equine Massage Awareness
PO Box 39003
RPO Billings Bridge
Ottawa
Ontario
K1H 1A1
Canada

Equine Sports Massage ITEC Diploma
Downs House Equine Rehabilitation
Combeleigh
Wheddon Cross
Minehead
Somerset
TA24 7AT

The London School of Shiatsu
Dugdale House
Santers Lane

Potters Bar
Hertfordshire
EN6 2BZ

Jack Meagher Institute
contact: Joanne Wilson
tel: (001) 978 456 9119 (USA)

Tteam and Ttouch Training
PO Box 3793
Santa Fe
NM 87501
USA

MASSAGE AIDS

Water Massage Boots
Sarah Williams Equine Therapy
Northfield Farmhouse
Thornton Curtis
Ulceby
DN39 6XW

Sore No More
Equine America
7 Lawson Hunt Business Park
Broadbridge Heath
West Sussex
RH12 3JR

LEGAL

Equine Lawyers Association
PO Box 23
Brigg
Lincolnshire
DN20 8TN

Bibliography

ACUPRESSURE AND ACUPUNCTURE

Foreign Language Press (Beijing, China), *Essentials of Chinese Acupuncture*

Giniaux, *Soulagez votre Cheval aux Doights* (ISBN 2828902579)

Jarmey, Chris, *Principles of Shiatsu* (ISBN 0722533624)

Kaptchuk, Ted, *Chinese Medicine – The Web That Has No Weaver* (ISBN 0091532310)

Kilde and Kung, *Veterinary Acupuncture* (ISBN 081227721X)

Lis-Balchin, Maria, *Aroma Science* (ISBN 1899308105)

Schon, Allen, *Veterinary Acupuncture – Ancient Art to Modern Medicine* (ISBN 032300945X)

Zidonis, Soderberg and Snow, *Equine Acupressure* (ISBN 0964598213)

MASSAGE

Chaitow, Leon, *Modern Neuromuscular Techniques* (ISBN 0443052980)

Holey and Cook, *Therapeutic Massage* (ISBN 0702019232)

Meagher, Jack, *Beating Muscle Injuries for Horses*

Tellington-Jones, *Improve Your Horse's Well-Being* (ISBN 1872119182)

ANATOMY AND NEUROANATOMY

Bach and Clayton, *Equine Locomotion* (ISBN 070202483X)

Budras, Sack and Rock, *Anatomy of the Horse* (ISBN 0723419213)

De Lahunter, *Veterinary Neuroanatomy and Clinical Neurology* (ISBN 0721630294)

Goody, *Horse Anatomy* (ISBN 0851312306)

Metzler, *Biochemistry – The Chemical Reactions of Living Cells* (ISBN 0124925308)

von Rautenfeld, Dr Berens, 'Manuelle Lymphdrainage beim Pferd' (*Pferdeheikunde* 16, Jan/Feb 2000)

Seiferle, *Nervensystem Sinnesorgane Endokrine Drusen*

Sissons and Grossman, *The Anatomy of Domestic Animals* Vol. 1 (ISBN 0721641024)

Sissons and Grossman, *The Anatomy of Domestic Animals* Vol. 2 (ISBN 0721641075)

Steen, Montagu, *Anatomy and Physiology,* Vol. 2 (ISBN 1389001392)

RIDER BALANCE

von Deitz, *Balance in der Bewegung* (ISBN 3885422581)

Loch, *The Classical Seat* (ISBN 0044401779)

Museler, *Riding Logic* (ISBN 0413532208)

Swift, *Centred Riding* (ISBN 0312127340)

PERIODICALS

The Holistic Horse
20 Prospect Avenue
Ardsley
NY 10502
USA

Natural Horse
PO Box 10
Holtwood
PA 17532
USA

Index